# About Nutrition

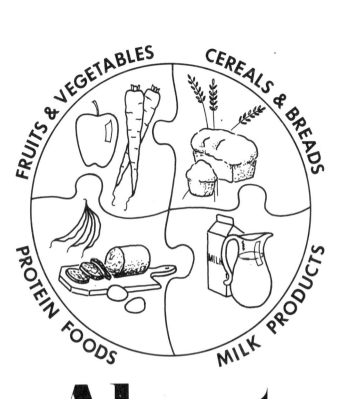

# About Nutrition

**By the Seventh-day Adventist Dietetic Association**

*Authors*
Alice G. Marsh, M.S., R.D.
Dorothy Christensen, M.S., R.D.
Rose G. Stoia, B.S., R.D.
Sylvia M. Fagal, M.S., R.D.

*Coordinator*
Darlene R. Schmitz, B.S., R.D.

Southern Publishing Association, Nashville, Tennessee

This book was
Edited by Richard W. Coffen
Designed by Dean Tucker

Cover painting by Ronald Hester

Text set in 11/13 Fairfield
Printed on Sorg Hi Bulk Offset
Cover stock: Springhill Gloss Bristol

Offset in U.S.A.

# Acknowledgments

I would like to thank the authors of this book, particularly Alice G. Marsh, who contributed greatly from her background of experience and original research in the field of nutrition and created the preschool puzzle concept to illustrate the Four Food Groups.

I acknowledge Royalynn B. Case, M.S., R.D., who worked with the authors during the first writing of the manuscript; Clinton A. Wall, B.S., R.D., for the book title, ABOUT NUTRITION, and for his contribution in developing the philosophy and organization of the book; and Barbara J. Myers, M.S., R.D., for assistance during the final stages of writing. I also express appreciation to the Seventh-day Adventist Dietetic Association Publication Committee, Ruth Little Carey, Ph.D., R.D., Chairman; Kathleen K. Zolber, Ph.D., R.D.; Irma B. Vyhmeister, M.S., R.D.; Ardis S. Beckner, M.S., R.D., for evaluation of material presented and for suggestions given.

Finally, I thank Frank Knittel, Ph.D., Hedwig Jemison, Shirley C. Johnson, and Charlene Scott for reading the manuscript.

DARLENE R. SCHMITZ,
*Registered Dietitian*

# Preface

Utilizing recent advances in science and nutrition research, the Seventh-day Adventist Dietetic Association has prepared this volume written in four sections:

*Section I* sets the theme for the entire book, using the Four Food Groups as the basis for daily nutritional needs.

*Section II* guides those responsible for menu planning and food budgets to include the Four Food Groups wisely, and shows how to prepare food in the most appealing way, yet conserving the nutritional value.

*Section III* presents guidelines for adjusting the Four Food Groups to meet nutritional needs from childhood to old age, and discusses nutrition management during common illnesses.

*Section IV* helps the reader see how the facts presented throughout the text establish a sound program of nutrition, using familiar foods available in local markets, and shows the dangers of fad diets with limited food selection.

This book presents the lacto-ovo-vegetarian diet as adequate within the framework of the Four Food Groups. In this diet, milk (lacto), eggs (ovo), and plant sources (vegetarian) provide the protein, and a variety of fruits, vegetables, grains, and nuts furnish other required nutrients. Proteins from a plant source contain unsaturated fat and have less total fat. Thus, the book shows the advantage of a lacto-ovo-vegetarian diet during a century when heart diseases continue to increase.

The 1968 Recommended Dietary Allowances have been used as a basis to verify the adequacy of a lacto-ovo-vegetarian diet. For an accurate and convenient dietary analysis reference, readers should obtain Home and Garden Bulletin No. 72 from the United States Department of Agriculture, Superintendent of Documents, U.S. Government Printing Office, Washington, D.C. 20402.

# Table of Contents

## SECTION I

## Nuggets of Knowledge on Nutrients

Chapter 1
# FOUR FOOD GROUPS FIT

The happiest discovery about nutrition is that good nutrition results from eating ordinary foods. We must learn how to group foods, how much to eat, and how to properly prepare food; and, as in other sciences and arts, an endless amount of knowledge abounds. Such a vast and vital study necessitates a working knowledge for all. Not only must the nonscientist have the needed information available to him, but also the nutritional scientist must have a simple device to apply in everyday living. Everyone needs an easy-to-follow, everyday guide for the life-or-death matter of correct eating.

Everyone bears the responsibility for food selection, preservation, preparation, and consumption, and it does not go away. Although the homemaker and the food service administrator assume the greater share of the burden, the individual consumer makes the final decision as to how much good nutrition, good art, good fun, and good living mix with the food he eats.

The attitudes associated with choosing daily food should not center entirely around the inquiry, "What do I like?" but rather, "Which foods will give the best possible body function and up-keep for today?" The person who has learned to like good foods discovers that the very foods he likes best fit into a plan assuring good nutrition.

Conveniently, good nutrition possesses a "least common denominator" known as the "Four Food Groups," which resembles a simple preschool puzzle. Like all puzzles, they make sense when put together, but they do not go together unless each piece fits exactly into its place. One piece cannot replace another.

The Four Food Groups idea has succeeded as a guide for daily diet planning because it encompasses all foods that nature provides. Besides this, the foods of most world cultures (except in areas where civilization exceeds food acquisition) fit into this basic plan. Thus the individual choosing his food can select any of the foods available to him—from all fruits and vegetables, from all cereals and breads, from all foods that contribute liberally to the body's need for protein, from all dairy products. One survey revealed the abundance of foods fitting into the plan by discovering sixty-six varieties of fresh, fresh frozen, and canned vegetables available the year around in one Midwestern small-town area. Although foods fit into but four groups, the selection in each group is amazingly abundant.

Four servings each day from the first two groups and two servings each day from the second two groups constitute the daily minimum from the Four Food Groups.

Fruit and Vegetable Group ............................ 4 servings
    1 serving of which provides a good source of vitamin C
        (Citrus fruit, tomatoes, or fresh raw vegetables)
    1 serving of which provides a good source of vitamin A
        (A very dark green or yellow vegetable)
Cereal and Bread Group ............................ 4 servings
    (Whole grain or enriched)
Protein Group ---------------------------------- 2 servings
Milk Group ---------------------------------- 2 servings

**The Food Groups Make a Nutritional Puzzle Fit**

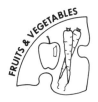

The fruit and vegetable group includes an almost endless variety of foods a parent should introduce to every child early in life when he learns and accepts various tastes. The body converts certain carotenes into vitamin A. One serving of cooked or raw carrots, broccoli, yellow squash or pumpkin, rutabaga, or any of the very green "greens" assures enough vitamin A. Interestingly, a food may play a double role in the menu; for instance, pumpkin pie doubles for a yellow vegetable; sweet potatoes serve as both the starchy vegetable and the food with vitamin A value. Most vegetable juices served as a beverage also abound in potential vitamin A. When you use a lesser green or yellow vegetable such as peas, green or wax beans, asparagus, or lima beans, which have less vitamin A value, select a very green or yellow vegetable the next day.

One certain cereal usually predominates in the diet of each distinct world culture. In countries composed of various old cultures, the citizens tend toward better nourishment when they have learned to like a variety of cereal grains served in many ways. The use of various cereal grains not only improves nutrition but also adds social interest to everyday eating. Cereal grains, depended upon as the primary dietary staple, are relatively inexpensive, available, and satisfying—a bland food that combines well with colorful and highly flavorful foods. For the most part, select cereals and breads from whole grains, or nearly whole grains. Many people advisably use cereals and flours with the roughest outer hull milled off or else finely milled whole-grain flour. All refined flour and cereal used should be enriched. Probably a good rule for meal planning is: Use at least half of the cereal and breads as whole grain.

15

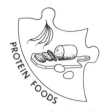

The protein food group includes the large variety of legumes (mature beans and peas), eggs and egg dishes, gluten (wheat protein), soy products, and many tasty combinations. Whether produced at home or by food companies, these foods make excellent vegetable protein meat analogues.* Nuts and nut butters contribute some protein to the diet, but because with few exceptions nuts have more fat than any other nutrient, they are not major contributors of protein in a well-managed diet. In the nonvegetarian diet, lean meat, fish, and fowl fit in this group.

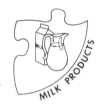

Milk and milk products contribute liberally to the protein needs of the body, but a separate milk group is needed to include certain nutrients the other food groups—including other protein foods—do not abundantly provide. The milk group assures calcium, riboflavin, and vitamin B12. Milk also efficiently provides proteins that supplement less effective proteins in other foods. Since milk is nutritionally efficient, include it in some form at each meal. You can serve whole milk, 2 percent fat milk, evaporated milk, skim milk (fluid, evaporated, or reconstituted dry), buttermilk, yogurt, or chocolate milk. Consider the latter a dessert and serve very moderately. Fortified soybean milk-type beverages adequately substitute for milk, or may be used as a milk alter-

*Meat analogues are made by General Foods Corporation, White Plains, New York; Loma Linda Foods, La Sierra, California; Worthington Foods, Incorporated, Worthington, Ohio, subsidiary to Miles Laboratories, Elkhart, Indiana.

nate. Cheese may contribute either as a milk group serving or as a serving in the protein group.

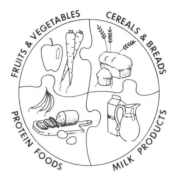

With the "least common denominator" of good nutrition fitted together, everyone is entitled to stack the pieces to make the daily diet fit his personal food requirements. To supply the needs of different ages and conditions, the Four Food Groups puzzle takes on a third dimension by stacking. Each piece added to the stack represents a serving.

**Stacking the Food Groups Fits Various People's Requirements**

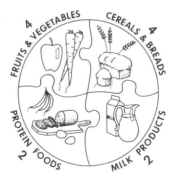

*First of all* everyone needs each of the four pieces of the food groups stacked in the number indicated to represent the number of servings—4, 4, 2, 2. ("Food for Fitness: A Daily Food Guide," United States Department of Agriculture, Agricultural Research Service.) This plan makes a good low-calorie diet for adults, since food choices from the Four Food Groups plan alone usually do not exceed 1,200 calories. If skim milk replaces whole milk, the plan constitutes a very satisfactory diet of approximately 1,000 calories. To add calories, a person should use more fruits, vegetables, and cereals, with limited amounts of "additions." (See page 20.) Maintenance of proper weight for each individual determines the amount of "additions" to use.

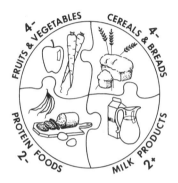

*Little folks* need the same foods as adults, but in small or even tiny servings. Add an extra milk serving if it does not cause the young child to exclude foods of the other groups.

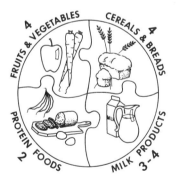

*School-age youngsters* may eat as much or more than their parents, plus extra milk. The amounts they require vary from child to child and for the same child from day to day. Providing enough of the proper food throughout the child's development is the parent's responsibility. The normal child who has learned to like good food usually eats the right amount for himself with a reasonable amount of "additions." (See page 20.)

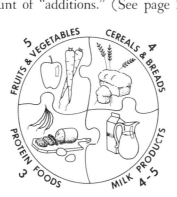

*Teen-agers* and even pre-teens necessitate a third serving of protein food, an extra vitamin C food, and two or three extra servings of milk. Supply more energy foods, if needed, with others of the Four Food Groups foods, especially whole-grain cereal and bread selections. Select "additions" carefully to add energy food and to contribute to the abundance of nutrients demanded by teen's growth and development. Teen treats and snacks should contribute protein, minerals, and vitamins as well as calories.

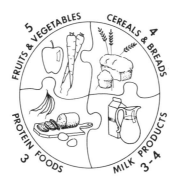

*Pregnancy's* extra nutritional requirements are met, first of all, by the woman's lifetime of good nutrition. Studies show that the years of good nutrition before conception as well as during pregnancy provide the greatest assurance of proper development of the new life. Added to her normal diet, she needs one extra serving each of milk, a vitamin C food, and a protein food. As the demand of the developing child increases, the pregnant woman's nutritional puzzle acquires a third dimension of 5, 4, 3, 3-4, respectively, of fruits and vegetables for the extra servings of vitamin C food, cereals and breads, protein foods, and milk.

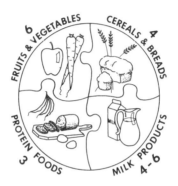

The lactating woman calls for further additions to the diet—from two to four extra servings of milk (this can be skim milk), two extra servings of a vitamin C food, and one extra protein food. Thus her food servings stack a minimum of 6, 4, 3, 4-6, respectively, of fruits and vegetables, cereals and breads, protein foods, and milk.

**Additions: A Few for Everyone—Very Little for Some**

Common "additions" to the Four Food Groups are fats and sweets, which must be used sparingly. These "additions" include spreads, cooking fats, salad dressings, seed oils, olives, avocados, nuts, jellies and jams, syrups, honey, and sugars. When restricting your calories, use these "additions" sparingly—if at all—except for a minimum daily inclusion of approximately two teaspoons of a seed oil, such as corn oil. However, do not overlook the important addition of water. While adding zero calories, water is important to all functions of the body and vital to good nutrition.

Choose it as a between-meal "snack" frequently during the day.

The good homemaker or the trained food service director provides each day the foods that complete the puzzle of the Four Food Groups and excludes no food from the pool of selections but utilizes foods of all seasons, tapping nature's storehouse each day. Complicated meals or a narrow selection need not exist. Nutrition for every individual can be perfect.

Notice the following day's menu of typical foods selected from the Four Food Groups. The "additions" add appeal and satisfaction, enabling the individual to select sufficient total calories.

### Breakfast

Orange Slices
Rolled Oats
Scrambled Egg          White Enriched Toast
Milk

### Dinner

Baked Brown Beans
Stuffed Baked Potato          Buttered Cauliflower
Lettuce and Tomato Salad
Whole-wheat Rolls          Soft-type Margarine*
Ice Cream With Sweet Wafers
Hot Cereal Drink Made With Milk

### Supper or Lunch

Cream of Mushroom Soup
Whole-wheat Wafers
Peanut Butter Sandwiches          Stewed Dried Apricots
Milk

It is impractical and unnecessary to calculate the major nutrients in every day's meals. Utilization of the Four Food Groups as a guide in menu making automatically assures their presence almost without exception.

---

*Liquid seed oil as the first or second stated ingredient.

For those who like to study figures, Table 1 calculates the menu for its calorie (kcal or large calorie) content and for eight nutrients. It compares the totals of each with the recommended dietary allowances for men and for women suggested by the Food and Nutrition Board of the National Research Council. (*Recommended Dietary Allowances,* Seventh Edition, National Academy of Sciences, 1968.) It bases the recommendations on the average growth pattern of North Americans.

The choices from the Four Food Groups given in Table 1, page 25, furnish 1,186 calories. The "additions" on page 26 increase the total calories to 2,036. Thus, the menu basically supplies all nutritional requirements, except that most men require more food for sufficient calories (energy), and women may need more iron, which additional vegetables, fruits, and whole grains would provide.

The Four Food Groups form the basis of good food selection for the family. Individual family members can adapt to their specific dietary needs by availing themselves of more food selections and by making food "additions" wisely. Find the recommended dietary allowances for specific sex and age groups on pages 178, 179.

Much flexibility must be allowed for individuals to choose amounts of food. Some people are normally "easy keepers" by efficiently using nutrients. Other people are not. Some may need additional amounts of most nutrients, while others need additional amounts of only one or two. Although the needs of individuals vary, people of the same age, sex, and within a moderate size range, require surprisingly similar amounts of protein, minerals, and vitamins.

Individual teen-age requirements vary the most. Nature intends some young persons to become larger than average in bone structure—some smaller. Some acquire their full growth early in the teen years—some later—even into the early twenties. Appetite, if based on good food habits, is usually a good guide for the amounts of food needed.

The child who has furnished for him foods ample in nutritional factors, attractively yet simply served, and at regular meal intervals, is indeed fortunate. Parents should provide this advantage for their child until he can capably assume the responsibility for himself.

Using the Four Food Groups as a simple everyday guide, the individual homemaker or food service director then daily chooses her menu from the hundreds of available foods. Even so, those foods most available and best liked constitute often-repeated old favorites. Table 1 illustrates a day's choice of economical foods from the four groups, with the addition of other foods to give sufficient calories and satisfaction to the meal, as well as a reasonable amount of well-chosen fat.

The choices, with a total calorie value of 2,036, correctly approximate the caloric needs for many active women but fall below the needs of the average man. Smaller or larger servings and more or less of additional foods adjust calories to the needs of each person, for the calorie criterion is to maintain correct weight. Little children eat less; older children and teen-agers eat more and larger servings. However, children and teen-agers, as well as adults, should not gain excess weight.

Many foods amply provide protein both in quantity and quality, although they usually cost more than other foods. The food choices used in the example furnish both inexpensive and highly adequate protein. If a diet provides too high a calorie level, cut cost and calories by replacing some or all of the milk with reconstituted, nonfat dry milk.

The calcium is adequate for all members of the family except in the event of rapid growth, but additional servings of the milk group care for these conditions.

Some may consider iron the problem nutrient, since it may appear that food is inadequate in iron and hence iron medication must supplement the diet. The calculated diet furnishes 14.3 milligrams of iron—more than a man requires. This amount of iron may fall below the requirement for some women, depending upon the amounts of menstrual blood loss. Actually, most drinking water and other accidental sources contain enough iron to supplement the iron in adequate food choices. It is unlikely that any normal person will become anemic if he properly chooses from the Four Food Groups. Iron pills or other medication can lead to intestinal irritation and to iron "overload." Do not give iron medication to children or adults unless a physician directs, and then only for the time indicated.

Vitamin A abounds. In fact, a deep green or yellow vegetable chosen every other day and alternating with less colorful vegetables still provides an abundance of this vitamin.

When one's food furnishes the three B vitamins (thiamine, riboflavin, and niacin) and sufficient high biologic protein (see chapters 3 and 5), all the other B vitamins are well supplied. Some foods contain preformed niacin; protein supplies the rest. The body can convert tryptophan, an essential amino acid (see chapter 3), into niacin when sufficient protein is available to the body. In the choice of foods in Table 1 the food directly supplies approximately half of the niacin, while the ample supply of high biologic protein furnishes the other half.

No problem exists regarding ascorbic acid when you include a serving of a citrus food. Many other foods form equally good sources of the vitamin, but never mistakenly assume that just any fruit, fruit drink, or fruitlike drink supplies it. (See Table 7, pages 68 and 69, for vitamin C food sources.)

Within the structure of the Four Food Groups make any other choices from the endless variety of foods available. All regular foods fit into a group, and many other choices are equally satisfactory. If calculated, each set of choices would reveal the same two facts: (1) food choices of the Four Food Groups can be made from all good foods; (2) these choices lead to excellent nutrition for all members of the family.

Table 1   The Nutrient Content of Foods Selected From the Four Food Groups

| Food | Common Measure | Wt. in Grams | Calories kcal | Protein gm. | Calcium mg. | Iron mg. | Vit. A I.U. | Thiamine mg. | Riboflavin mg. | Niacin mg. | Ascorbic Acid mg. |
|---|---|---|---|---|---|---|---|---|---|---|---|
| **Fruit and Vegetable Group** | | | | | | | | | | | |
| Potato, baked | 1 medium | 100 | 90 | 3 | 9 | .7 | trace | .10 | .04 | 1.7 | 20 |
| Cauliflower | 1 cup | 120 | 25 | 3 | 25 | .8 | 70 | .11 | .10 | .7 | 66 |
| Orange | 3" diameter | 210 | 86 | 1 | 67 | .3 | 310 | .16 | .06 | .6 | 70 |
| Apricots, dried, uncooked | ¼ cup, 10 small halves | 38 | 98 | 2 | 25 | 2.0 | 4,088 | .0 | .06 | 1.2 | 5 |
| **Cereal and Bread Group** | | | | | | | | | | | |
| Rolled Oats, cooked | ⅔ cup | 157 | 87 | 3 | 14 | .9 | 0 | .13 | .03 | .2 | 0 |
| Bread, whole-grain | 2 slices | 46 | 110 | 4 | 46 | 1.0 | trace | .12 | .06 | 1.4 | trace |
| Bread, white enriched | 1 slice | 23 | 60 | 2 | 19 | .6 | trace | .06 | .05 | .6 | trace |
| **Protein Group** | | | | | | | | | | | |
| Beans, common varieties, cooked | 1 cup | 256 | 230 | 15 | 74 | 4.6 | trace | .13 | .10 | 1.5 | - - |
| Egg | 1 | 50 | 80 | 6 | 27 | 1.1 | 590 | .05 | .15 | trace | 0 |
| **Milk Group** | | | | | | | | | | | |
| Milk, whole | 2 cups | 488 | 320 | 18 | 576 | .2 | 700 | .16 | .84 | .2 | 4 |
| Totals from diet | | | 1,186 | 57 | 882 | 12.2 | 5,758 | 1.02 | 1.49 | 8.1 | 165 |
| Recommended allowance for a man: | | | 2,800 | 65 | 800 | 10 | 5,000 | 1.4 | 1.7 | 18 | 60 |
| for a woman: | | | 2,000 | 55 | 800 | 18 | 5,000 | 1.0 | 1.5 | 13 | 55 |

Table 1 (cont.)   Food Additions to the Four Food Groups to Complete a Typical Day's Diet

| Food | Common Measure | Wt. in Grams | Calories kcal | Protein gm. | Calcium mg. | Iron mg. | Vit. A I.U. | Thiamine mg. | Riboflavin mg. | Niacin mg. | Ascorbic Acid mg. |
|---|---|---|---|---|---|---|---|---|---|---|---|
| **Additions** | | | | | | | | | | | |
| Margarine, oil 1st ingredient | 1 tbsp. | 14 | 100 | tr | 3 | 0 | 460 | - - | - - | - - | 0 |
| Oil, corn | 1 tbsp. | 14 | 125 | 0 | 0 | 0 | - - | 0 | 0 | 0 | 0 |
| Mayonnaise | 1 tbsp. | 15 | 110 | tr | 3 | .1 | 40 | tr | .01 | tr | - - |
| Lettuce | 3 oz. | 85 | 9 | - - | 15 | .4 | 266 | .04 | .04 | .2 | 5 |
| Tomato | 1 med. | 150 | 35 | 2 | 20 | .8 | 1,350 | .10 | .06 | 1.0 | 34 |
| Cream of Mushroom Soup | ⅓ can | | 111 | 2 | 34 | .3 | 60 | .01 | .10 | 0.6 | - - |
| Peanut butter | 1 tbsp. | 16 | 95 | 4 | 9 | .3 | - - | .02 | .02 | 2.4 | 0 |
| Ice cream | ⅛ qt. | | 145 | 3 | 87 | - - | 370 | .03 | .13 | .1 | - - |
| Wafers, sweet | 2 small | | 120 | 1 | 9 | .2 | 20 | .01 | .01 | .1 | 0 |
| Total from 4 Food Groups | | | 1,186 | 57 | 882 | 12.2 | 5,758 | 1.02 | 1.49 | 8.1 | 165 |
| Food Groups Diet Additions | | | 850 | 12 | 180 | 2.1 | 2,566 | .21 | .37 | 4.4 | 39 |
| Total for day's selections | | | 2,036 | 69 | 1,062 | 14.3 | 8,324 | 1.23 | 1.86 | 12.5 | 204 |

From tryptophan of protein*        11.5

24.0

*Niacin from its precursor, tryptophan.

Chapter 2
# BODY'S BIG BUSINESS

Envision the Four Food Groups as four large packages of nutrients. You interlock the four large pieces of this simple food puzzle and thus provide all units needed for building and maintaining each cell of the body. As body cells receive the materials given them by way of food, they become individual factories making and putting together puzzle pieces which we can liken to the most intricate puzzle of one thousand pieces or more. The imagination can understand only with difficulty that nutrition is both as simple as the Four Food Groups, and at the same time as complex as the functions of a single body cell.

The body can properly build and maintain itself only if correct materials are available when needed. A body cell, the unit of body structure, requires at least fifty nutrients. With these nutrient units the cell makes its own structure, as well as its own hundreds of specific enzymes and coenzymes that aid the individual cell's use of nutrients. Certain cells of glands also produce necessary hormones that effectively regulate vital body functions. The body cells also make many other complex substances from the materials supplied by food, water, and air.

### Metabolism

The term "metabolism" encompasses all functions of cells and their organizations (tissues and organs). *Anabolism,* the building of complex substances by cells, balances *catabolism,* the breaking down of complex substances for energy utilization and excretion of end products of metabolism. For most adults, anabolism and catabolism are equal in effect. However, in growth,

27

pregnancy, lactation, and actual body building, the processes of anabolism are greater than those of catabolism, whereas in acute illnesses, loss of weight, and destructive conditions due to hormone imbalance, catabolism exceeds anabolism. In health, and with proper eating habits and exercise, metabolism amazingly holds itself in continuous balance and often does so for a lifetime.

### The Nutrients and Their Functions

Most of the nutrients serve more than one function, and all are essential and available from foods of the Four Food Groups. We can list their functions under the following categories:

Nutrients That Build and Maintain Body Cells
  Protein                     Mineral elements
  Water                       Fats
  Carbohydrates

Nutrients That Regulate Body Functions
  Water                   Vitamins
  Mineral elements    Carbohydrates, including cellulose

Nutrients That Provide Energy
  Carbohydrates                Fats
    (starches and sugars)      Proteins

### The Reconstruction of Food

Food preparation begins in the kitchen. Many foods can be served raw, others raw or cooked, while many must be cooked before certain nutrients are available and acceptable to the body. Good food preparation is both a science and an art and should capture the interest of every homemaker. First of all, learn those basic procedures assuring the best use of food without the inclusion of excess calories or loss of important nutrients. Section II discusses such basic facts and procedures for the preparation of food and its service to individuals and families. Learning to use good procedures in preparation assures that food reaches the table in its best condition for nourishing the body as well as pleasing and satisfying the diners.

Food preparation should ensure:

Food clean and safe.
Proteins in their most available form.
Starches available to digestive enzymes.
Fats unharmed chemically and not soaked into starches.
Minerals retained and available.
Vitamins retained.
Cellulose softer.
Natural color retained.
Flavor retained and enhanced.
Odor pleasant and provocative to digestive response (makes the mouth water).
Food available in an attractive setting (even in a lunch box on the job).

Digestion actually continues food preparation in the gastrointestinal tract. The digestive processes break down the food eaten into the nutrients suitable for entry into the bloodstream, and then and there the metabolic processes begin.

Chewing prepares food for digestion in the digestive tract, although food undergoes slight digestion in the mouth. Fortunately, you cannot swallow food easily until you chew it reasonably well, mixing it with saliva, which begins starch digestion. The stomach mixes the food with more digestive juices until it becomes quite liquid. Starches continue to digest until the contents become acid with hydrochloric acid; pepsin begins digesting protein, and rennin curds casein (a protein of milk). The fats that are already separated in particles (emulsified) may digest to some extent in the stomach also.

Most digestion occurs in the small intestine. In the presence of bile, digestive enzymes from the pancreas and the intestinal wall reduce foods to their digestive end products:

Carbohydrates to the single sugars (glucose, fructose, and galactose).
Fats to fatty acids and glycerol (glycerine).
Proteins to their building block units (amino acids).

Some food material is not intended for digestion and absorption. Cellulose, or fiber, mainly stimulates the activity of the intestinal tract. The intestine normally excretes about 2 percent of the carbohydrate, 5 percent of the fat, 8 percent of the protein of the typical mixed diet, the cellulose, and a small amount of water.

Absorption of nutrients takes place along the entire length of the small intestine. Not passively or casually, but actively, complex substances in the stomach and chemical forces in the whole digestive tract transport the nutrients across the intestinal barrier. For a number of nutrients, absorption occurs only in specified areas of the tract. Water-soluble nutrients entering the cells lining the digestive tract are transferred to blood capillaries and carried to larger and larger blood vessels, then on to the liver. Most of the fat-soluble nutrients go from digestive tract cells into the lymph, and thus indirectly into the bloodstream.

For proper nourishment, furnish the body daily with the foods of the Four Food Groups. Given the "raw material," the body cares for all the intricate details involved in the acts of nutrition. Simple consideration for nutritional needs by planning around the Four Food Groups—

1. Gives sufficient nutrients (except perhaps calories or certain trace nutrients lacking in local soil or water, such as iodine and fluorine).

2. Serves as a food guide for all ages above infancy, with modification of amounts.

3. Provides the protein requirement both in quantity and quality, thus giving specific amino acids for all structures of the body, including those needed to make highly specialized substances, such as enzymes, hormones, and antibodies.

4. Furnishes adequately the less understood nutrients in biologically adequate amounts, such as vitamin $B_{12}$, the pyridoxines, folic acid, and certain trace minerals.

5. Automatically maintains the acid and base balance of the body.

6. Gives the correct kind and amount of fiber in the diet.

7. Adequately supplies calcium and riboflavin which can be lacking when meat constitutes the main protein food and takes the place of both the protein and milk group.

8. Makes it possible to select from the hundreds of varieties of food, thus eliminating no food nature provides.

9. Combines nutrients that facilitate assimilation and utilization of foods.

10. Gives opportunity to regulate the amount and kind of additional selected fats used.

11. Recognizes bland foods which make the diet more tolerable and provide a basis for enjoyment of colorful and flavorful foods.

12. Leaves no place for faddishness and misinformation of foods.

13. Adapts the lacto-ovo-vegetable protein diet, which provides an excellent plan for food selection.

14. Uses a simple tool in food selection of 4-4-2-2 in terms of servings for each respective group of foods.

15. Furnishes good nutrition with easily procured, ordinary foods in simple, programmed selection that practically assures good nutrition without threat of overnutrition or imbalance of nutrients.

16. Presents a dietary plan adaptable to people and their native foods throughout the world.

One can only wonder how a simple plan in food selection can assure so much in nutritional science and functional body chemistry!

From the gastrointestinal tract, the nutrients directly or indirectly issue continuously into the blood. Immediately these vital materials go to work nourishing every cell of the body. The person interested in this continuous process refers to the Four Food Groups in planning daily meals, and each day chooses a different selection of foods. Thus he utilizes all foods, good nutrition continues, and good fellowship centers around mealtime.

Chapter 3

## THE FIRE OF LIFE

*Fire,* usually a terrifying word, is a welcome one in terms of body metabolism, although scientists temper the word by substituting the term "oxidation." After using carbohydrates, fats, and proteins for building and storage, the body utilizes them for energy. This process requires a "slow burn" as the carbon materials of these nutrients combine with oxygen. The hemoglobin (a protein-iron complex) in the red blood cells carries oxygen from the lungs and releases it near every cell of the body, which accepts nutrients from the blood for fuel. The oxidation of the three nutrients releases energy, gives the body power to work, and produces heat as a by-product. The body's temperature remains at approximately 98.6 degrees Fahrenheit, and the person lives—active and capable of great potential in physical and mental work.

### The Carbohydrates

Green plants use energy from the sun, water from the soil, and carbon dioxide from the air to produce sugars and starches, which provide man with the major source of his energy requirement. In the United States, carbohydrate furnishes about half of the energy food of the diet. In many parts of the world, as much as four fifths of the total calories come from the starches of cereal seeds. Cereals and sugars form an acceptable, inexpensive, wholesome, and adaptable basis for other food inclusions.

Saccharide (sugar) units, composing all starches and sugars, are built by the plant in the following forms:

32

| Sugar Units | Examples | Some Food Sources |
|---|---|---|
| Monosaccharides (single sugars) | Glucose (dextrose) | Many fruits and vegetables, honey, corn syrup |
| | Fructose (levulose) | Many fruits and vegetables, honey, corn syrup |
| | Galactose | Does not occur except as milk sugar (lactose) is digested |
| Disaccharides (two sugar units) | Sucrose | Cane, beet, maple, fruits, and vegetables |
| | Maltose | From malting of cereal grains |
| | Lactose | Milk sugar, the only carbohydrate of milk |
| Polysaccharides (many sugar units) | Dextrin | Partially digested starches |
| | Cellulose | Fiber of fruits and vegetables, bran, coat of cereal grains |
| | Glycogen | Animal starch, in liver and muscles |

For every two units of a single sugar (monosaccharide), the plant takes out two hydrogen and one oxygen (one water molecule) molecules and bonds the two monosaccharides into one double sugar (disaccharide). As this process continues to add saccharide unit after saccharide unit, it forms large carbohydrate molecules such as starches. Thus the starchy seed or root can store potential energy for human use in a small space and in a form that offers good keeping qualities.

Eating these storehouses of energy reverses the chemical process occurring in the plant. Digestive juices furnish the water plus the specific enzymes to facilitate the process of adding water at the juncture of each two sugar units. Hence, the saccharide units split into monosaccharides as the food reaches certain absorptive areas of the small intestine.

Do not think, however, that eating simple sugars in the first place eases metabolism. First, starches come to us by nature mixed with small but important amounts of proteins and fats, small to liberal amounts of various minerals, vitamins, and cellulose, and many of the nutrients needed for their proper use and metabolism. To eat the simple or double sugars or the pure starches exclusively would lead to the inclusion of energy food only with little of the equally important nutrients. Second, nature does not intend that we have much sugar in the diet. Not only do man and nature tend to highly refine the distinct sugars, thus giving little more than calories, but digestion of starches in foods supplies energy food to the blood rather slowly over a continuous and longer period of time. Sugars ready for absorption at once oversupply the blood as well as the metabolic facilities of the body as they work to store the sugar in the form of body starch. As a homey example, the family may like a decorative wood carrier filled with wood sitting by the fireplace, but they prefer to store the cords of wood elsewhere than in the living room. The large starch molecules tend to serve as reserve fuel which does not disturb the housekeeping (metabolism) of the body. Sugars, on the other hand, tend to be demanding at both the absorptive facilities and metabolic sites. Therefore, take most of your carbohydrate in the form of large molecules (starch). Following the Four Food Groups as a guide in meal planning automatically accomplishes this feat, providing you use additional sweet foods in moderation.

Starches and sugars are friendly nutrients and the greatest supporters of the power to do work. Since misinformation regarding these nutrients runs rampant, chapter 17 discusses common facts and fallacies regarding starches and sugars, as well as giving a correct understanding of their often mistaken role.

Since some persons should use less than the full amount of the bran portion of cereals, milled flours are commonly used. However, since the processing destroys some nutrients, the Food and Drug Administration allows *enrichment* of cereals and flours by the addition of thiamine, riboflavin, niacin, and iron. In fact, more than half the states require such enrichment, and the other states voluntarily enrich bread and flour. Enriched flour, although nutritionally preferred over unenriched flour, does not contain all the nutrients lost in milling. However, through this nutritional health plan, enriched bread compares favorably with whole-wheat bread in nutritive value, in calories, protein, calcium, iron, and in B vitamins that other foods are not apt to replace.

Carbohydrates make up the nutrients used in the greatest quantity by the body; choose them mainly from whole food sources and for the most part in the form of large molecules (the starches).

**Fats**

The word *fat* conveys mixed interpretations and feelings to most people—rich, good, plenty versus unwanted, greasy, inferior. Fat is needed—is desirable—and deserves most careful consideration as a nutrient.

To make a fat molecule, three fatty acids of various length carbon chains (four to twenty-four carbon atoms) unite with the three alcohol units of a glycerol (glycerine) molecule. At each of the three points of union one water molecule is taken out. Fats can vary in nature greatly because of the many possible lengths of the carbon chain. Variation also exists in the number of places where the bonds may be doubled between carbon molecules rather than hold the greatest possible number of hydrogen atoms.

At this point, we can profitably clarify a number of terms commonly heard in discussions regarding dietary fats. All *fats* are made of three *fatty acids* and one glycerol. *Saturated* fatty acids are composed of carbon chains with no double bonds between carbons and with all carbon atoms "saturated" with as many hydrogen atoms as they can hold. In the following diagram of a portion of a saturated fatty acid, C signifies carbon, H signifies hydrogen, and O, oxygen:

$$-\overset{\displaystyle H}{\underset{\displaystyle H}{\overset{\displaystyle |}{\underset{\displaystyle |}{C}}}}-\overset{\displaystyle H}{\underset{\displaystyle H}{\overset{\displaystyle |}{\underset{\displaystyle |}{C}}}}-\overset{\displaystyle H}{\underset{\displaystyle H}{\overset{\displaystyle |}{\underset{\displaystyle |}{C}}}}-\overset{\displaystyle H}{\underset{\displaystyle H}{\overset{\displaystyle |}{\underset{\displaystyle |}{C}}}}-\overset{\displaystyle H}{\underset{\displaystyle H}{\overset{\displaystyle |}{\underset{\displaystyle |}{C}}}}-\overset{\displaystyle H}{\underset{\displaystyle H}{\overset{\displaystyle |}{\underset{\displaystyle |}{C}}}}-\overset{\displaystyle H}{\underset{\displaystyle H}{\overset{\displaystyle |}{\underset{\displaystyle |}{C}}}}-\overset{\displaystyle H}{\underset{\displaystyle H}{\overset{\displaystyle |}{\underset{\displaystyle |}{C}}}}-\overset{\displaystyle H}{\underset{\displaystyle H}{\overset{\displaystyle |}{\underset{\displaystyle |}{C}}}}-\overset{\displaystyle O}{\overset{\displaystyle \|}{C}}-OH$$

*Unsaturated* fatty acids have double energy bonds linking the carbons. If there is but one point of unsaturation, it is called a *monounsaturated* fatty acid as the following portion of a fatty acid shows:

$$-\overset{H}{\underset{H}{C}}-\overset{H}{C}=\overset{H}{C}-\overset{H}{\underset{H}{C}}-\overset{H}{\underset{H}{C}}-\overset{H}{\underset{H}{C}}-\overset{H}{\underset{H}{C}}-\overset{H}{\underset{H}{C}}-\overset{H}{\underset{H}{C}}-\overset{O}{\overset{\|}{C}}-OH$$

If the carbon chain contains more than one point of un-saturation, it is called a *polyunsaturated* fatty acid:

$$-\overset{H}{\underset{H}{C}}-\overset{H}{\underset{H}{C}}-\overset{H}{\underset{H}{C}}-\overset{H}{C}=\overset{H}{C}-\overset{H}{C}=C=\overset{H}{C}-\overset{H}{\underset{H}{C}}-\overset{H}{\underset{H}{C}}-\overset{H}{\underset{H}{C}}-\overset{H}{\underset{H}{C}}-\overset{H}{\underset{H}{C}}-\overset{H}{\underset{H}{C}}-\overset{O}{\overset{\|}{C}}-OH$$

In a polyunsaturated fat, a high portion of polyunsaturated fatty acids makes up the fat. These fats tend to be oils at room temperature. One polyunsaturated fatty acid that is plentiful in seed oils—*linoleic acid*—is essential to good nutrition. An essential substance in nutrition must be obtained directly from food—the body must have this chemical structure but cannot reconstruct from similar structures.

Oils can be manufactured into a plastic or moldable solid fat for shortening, for cooking, and for margarines. During this process of *hydrogenation,* hydrogen molecules attach to some of the carbons held by double bonds, thus reducing the number of double bonds, making them single. As hydrogenation increases the saturation of a fat, it decreases the amount of linoleic acid in the oil and converts the oil into a fat that remains solid at room temperature. The following formula illustrates the process:

$$\underset{H}{\overset{H}{\underset{|}{\overset{|}{-C}}}} - \underset{}{\overset{H}{\overset{|}{C}}} = \underset{}{\overset{H}{\overset{|}{C}}} - \underset{H}{\overset{H}{\underset{|}{\overset{|}{C}}}} - + \ H_2 \longrightarrow \underset{H}{\overset{H}{\underset{|}{\overset{|}{-C}}}} - \underset{H}{\overset{H}{\underset{|}{\overset{|}{C}}}} - \underset{H}{\overset{H}{\underset{|}{\overset{|}{C}}}} - \underset{H}{\overset{H}{\underset{|}{\overset{|}{C}}}} -$$

As the saturation increases and the oil becomes solid, it melts at a higher temperature than it originally did.

Fats used as fuel are almost two and one-half times more concentrated than carbohydrates and proteins. While the carbohydrates and proteins each produce four calories of heat per gram (approximately one thirtieth of an ounce), the fats yield nine calories per gram. This means that fats yield the most energy of the three calorie-producing nutrients.

*Antioxidants* added to fats lengthen their keeping quality. Without this protection fats turn rancid quickly.

On the plus side of the ledger, the diet needs fats, since they are good fuel foods and carry essential fatty acids and fat-soluble vitamins. Some fat accompanying meals adds a feeling of satisfaction (satiety). Omit fats from the diet, and you will experience dissatisfaction (lack of satiety).

On the negative side, fats can quickly put too many calories in the diet, leading to overweight. Since most fats and oils contain few essential nutrients, use them in moderation as a refined food. Because fats add richness to other foods, making them more appealing to most appetites, one can easily overuse them.

As a result of habit and common use, many people prefer the solid fats. In certain food preparation techniques solid fats emulsify easily through other food ingredients and are less visible, yet these solid fats are naturally low in linoleic acid or are produced by hydrogenation with a resultant loss of the polyunsaturated fatty acids.

Associated with today's affluent society is an abundance of oils manufactured into a nonoily, plastic, or pliable shortening to favor the American cook's demand. Concurrent with this trend, not only does the average person eat too many fat calories, but the intake of linoleic acid is relatively low and an unfavorable picture of blood lipids (fats) has appeared. The greatest concern has centered around abnormally elevated blood serum cholesterol and triglyceride (fat) levels. Cholesterol, normally present and needed in all tissues of the body, is a type of solid alcohol related to fat. Blood serum triglyceride levels measure the actual pure fats in the blood. An abnormally high concentration of these substances has been associated with coronary heart attacks called *infarct* and other related conditions of circulatory deterioration.

While science offers no direct proof that a person will avoid early heart attacks by merely altering the amount and kind of fat in the diet, the indirect proof is overwhelming. *Atherosclerosis,* a slowly developing disease of the arteries, begins with a thickening of the inner lining of the blood vessels from one to many layers of cells. Then various materials, including cholesterol, are deposited, and the blood vessel area narrows; meanwhile the vessel walls lose their elasticity. Even three of the following "high risk factors" present in an individual indicate needed dietary control. Better still, dietary control early in life before certain of these factors develop may be of utmost value.

The "high risk factors":

> Men (more subject to heart attacks than women).
> Hereditary factors (follow family trends due to genetic differences).
> Little exercise.
> Inner stress.
> Elevated blood cholesterol level.
> High blood pressure.
> Overweight.
> Cigarette smoking.
> Excess coffee drinking.
> Insufficient sleep.

Dietary control includes lowering total dietary fat in the typical American diet. This diet often contains more than 45 to 55 percent of its calories in fat. A diet in which fat composes only 35 percent of the calories shows promise of better balance. Carefully select separated fats (oils) so that they include ample amounts of linoleic acid unchanged by hydrogenation. Maintain a certain relationship of polyunsaturated fats to saturated fats in the diet, but reserve the saturated fats to dairy and egg fats, for they carry other essential nutrients such as fat-soluble vitamins.

Figure 1 shows percentages of linoleic acid in a number of fats and oils of plant and animal origin. Careful study shows that animal fats as a whole contain less of this essential fatty acid than do some of the vegetable fats. Safflower, corn, soy, and cottonseed oils provide readily available supplies of linoleic acid. Margarines on the market today containing liquid seed oils have higher percentages of linoleic acid than the solid stick margarines indicated in Figure 1.

Strictly avoid the temptation to overuse even the desirable oils, but, for the most part, choose the little separated fat you do use from the oils that supply linoleic acid.

Also include in the diet some of the saturated short-chained fatty acids that carry fat-soluble nutrients. A limited number of eggs, some milk fat, or fortified margarine with liquid oil as the first or second stated ingredient enhances the diet and gives a balance of fatty acids. Although egg yolks contain high amounts of cholesterol, they carry substances which aid the body to properly utilize fats. Furthermore, some evidence indicates that the body does not absorb all dietary cholesterol. Some studies show that the body absorbs only one and one-half times the square root of the ingested (eaten) cholesterol. (See article by Ancel Keys, "Blood Lipids in Man—A Brief Review," in *Journal of the American Dietetic Association*, December, 1967.) Hence, it appears that a moderate cholesterol intake for the normal person is not undesirable, but a higher intake is not recommended.

A lacto-ovo-vegetable diet may contain, in one day, two cups of whole milk, a serving of creamed cottage cheese (or a small serving of American cheese), one egg, and one-eighth quart of ice cream. This choice of food gives approximately 350 milli-

Figure 1

Percent of linoleic acid in fats and oils of plant and animal origin. (From Coons, in the *Journal of the American Dietetic Association*, 34:242, 1958. Courtesy of the American Dietetic Association.)

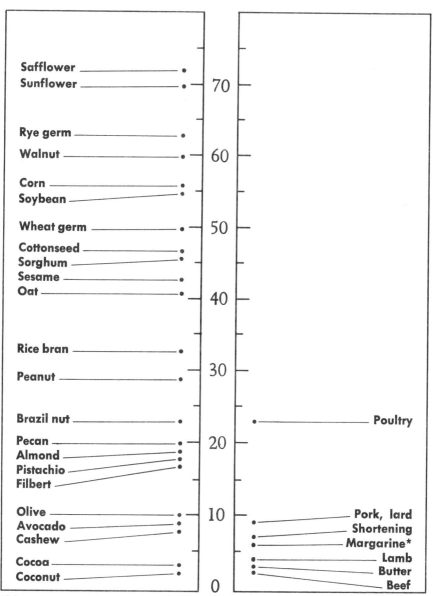

*Margarines containing liquid seed oils are higher in linoleic acid.

grams of cholesterol from food sources for the day—a low amount of dietary cholesterol. According to the theory of cholesterol absorption stated in the preceding paragraph, most people will absorb only nineteen milligrams of cholesterol from these dietary inclusions. Many diets that daily contain eggs and meats—especially organ meats—regularly include as much as 1,000 milligrams of cholesterol each day. Most people can handle efficiently the cholesterol of three to five eggs per week and will benefit from the nutrients provided.

Certain general recommendations have emerged from the study of types of fats and fatty acids in nutrition: (1) a diet containing 40 percent fat calories or more is undoubtedly too high in fat and should be lowered; (2) the daily diet should include some unhydrogenated (unhardened) seed oils; and (3) though highly saturated in nature, short carbon-chained fats in egg yolk and milk fat are of value in human nutrition when used moderately.

The ratio of polyunsaturated fat to saturated fat in the diet has arrested the interest of nutritionists and thoughtful lay persons. Both types of fatty acids are needed, but nutritionists generally agree that certain relationships between the two are more desirable than others.

Diets in which the fatty foods include only dairy and egg fats, meat fats from hard animal fats, and hydrogenated oils contain few polyunsaturates. With one gram of saturated fatty acids there may be only .04 gram of linoleic acid. (See Table 2, Diet No. 1.) When by altering these fat sources (Diet No. 2) to substitute a portion of the milk as nonfat milk, undiluted evaporated milk for cream, a beef-style soy protein food, corn oil, and soft margarine with liquid oil as the first or second stated ingredient, the ratio shifts decidedly. For one gram of saturated fatty acids there are three grams of linoleic acid. With the same number of servings of fat-containing foods, the total fat decreases 27 percent in the second diet. For those interested in these figures, careful food selection shifted the P/S ratio (the ratio of polyunsaturated fat in grams to saturated fat) of the day's diet (using

Table 2    The Polyunsaturate-Saturate Fatty Acids Ratio of a Day's Diet According to Four Different Fat Selections

| Food | Grams | Amount | Total Fat gm. | Saturated (total) gm. | Fatty Acids Unsaturated — Oleic gm. | Linoleic gm. | P/S Ratio |
|---|---|---|---|---|---|---|---|
| **Diet No. 1,** fat-containing foods | | | | | | | |
| Milk, whole | 732 | 3 cups | 27 | 15 | 9 | trace | |
| Egg | 50 | 1 | 6 | 2 | 3 | trace | |
| Butter | 28 | 2 tbsp. | 22 | 12 | 8 | trace | |
| Cream, 40% (whipping) | 30 | 2 tbsp. | 12 | 6 | 4 | trace | |
| Beef hamburger, regular | 85 | 3 oz. | 17 | 8 | 8 | trace | |
| Shortening | 25 | 2 tbsp. | 24 | 6 | 16 | 2 | 0.04 |
| **Totals** | | | **108** | **49** | **48** | **2** | |
| **Diet No. 2,** fat-containing foods | | | | | | | |
| Milk, whole | 244 | 1 cup | 9 | 5 | 3 | trace | |
| Milk, skim | 492 | 2 cups | trace | - - | - - | - - | |
| Egg | 50 | 1 | 6 | 2 | 3 | trace | |
| Evaporated milk, undiluted | 32 | 2 tbsp. | 2 | 1 | 1 | trace | |
| Beef-style soy product Prime slices—no gravy | 75 | 3 oz. | 5 | trace | 1 | 2 | |
| Oil, corn | 28 | 2 tbsp. | 28 | 2 | 8 | 14 | |

| | 28 | 2 tbsp. | 28 | 2 | 4 | 20 | 3.0 |
|---|---|---|---|---|---|---|---|
| Margarine, liquid seed oil first or second ingredient | 28 | 2 tbsp. | 28 | 2 | 4 | 20 | 3.0 |
| **Totals** | | | **78** | **12** | **20** | **36** | 0.61 |
| **Diet No. 3,** fat-containing foods | | | | | | | |
| Milk, whole | 732 | 3 cups | 27 | 15 | 9 | trace | |
| Egg | 50 | 1 | 6 | 2 | 3 | trace | |
| Margarine, liquid seed oil first or second ingredient | 28 | 2 tbsp. | 28 | 2 | 4 | 20 | |
| Cream, 40% | 30 | 2 tbsp. | 12 | 6 | 4 | trace | |
| Beef hamburger, lean | 85 | 3 oz. | 10 | 5 | 4 | trace | |
| Shortening | 25 | 2 tbsp. | 24 | 6 | 16 | 2 | |
| **Totals** | | | **107** | **36** | **40** | **22** | 0.61 |
| **Diet No. 4,** fat-containing foods | | | | | | | |
| Milk, whole | 732 | 3 cups | 27 | 15 | 9 | trace | |
| Egg | 50 | 1 | 6 | 2 | 3 | trace | |
| Margarine, liquid seed oil first or second ingredient | 28 | 2 tbsp. | 28 | 2 | 4 | 20 | |
| Cream, 40% | 30 | 2 tbsp. | 12 | 6 | 4 | trace | |
| Beef-style soy product | 75 | 3 oz. | 5 | trace | 1 | 2 | |
| O I, corn | 28 | 2 tbsp. | 28 | 2 | 8 | 14 | 1.33 |
| **Totals** | | | **106** | **27** | **29** | **36** | |

Table 3    The Polyunsaturate-Saturate Fatty Acid Ratio of a Day's Diet According to the Food Selections From the Four Food Groups in Table 1

| Food | Amount | Total Fat gm. | Saturated (total) gm. | Fatty Acids | | P/S Ratio |
|---|---|---|---|---|---|---|
| | | | | Unsaturated | | |
| | | | | Oleic gm. | Linoleic gm. | |
| Egg | 1 | 6 | 2 | 3 | trace | |
| Milk | 2 cups | 18 | 10 | 6 | trace | |
| Margarine, liquid seed oil first or second ingredient | 1 tbsp. | 14 | 1 | 2 | 10 | |
| Oil, corn | 1 tbsp. | 14 | 1 | 4 | 7 | |
| Mayonnaise | 1 tbsp. | 12 | 2 | 3 | 6 | |
| Cream of Mushroom soup—direct from can | ½ cup | 10 | 1 | 3 | 5 | |
| Peanut butter | 1 tbsp. | 8 | 2 | 4 | 2 | |
| Ice cream | ⅛ qt. | 9 | 5 | 3 | trace | 1.25 |
| **Totals** | | **91** | **24** | **28** | **30** | |

linoleic acid as the polyunsaturated fatty acid calculated) from 0.04 to 3.0.

The fat-containing foods of Diets Nos. 3 and 4 in Table 2 show how only two changes in the diet modified the fatty acid relationships. A beef-style soy product substitutes for the lean beef hamburger, and corn oil is used in place of shortening. For every gram of saturated fatty acid in Diet No. 3 there is 0.61 gram of linoleic acid. In Diet No. 4 the two food changes have resulted in 1.33 grams of linoleic acid to each gram of saturated fatty acids—a ratio change of 0.61 to 1.33.

Table 3 calculates the type of fat contained in the Four Food Groups given on page 25. The ratio of linoleic acid to saturated fatty acids is 1.25, which means there are 1.25 grams of linoleic acid for each gram of saturated fat. Although a P/S ratio of 3.0 may be prescribed in certain medical conditions, a ratio of approximately 1.0 may be desirable for regular dietary usage, which the thoughtful homemaker can easily accomplish.

With these facts in mind, carefully study Tables 2 and 3 so that you can incorporate the principles into meal planning. Careful food selection has accomplished three points worthy of consideration:

1. It decreases the total fat of a typical American diet.

2. It increases the relationship of linoleic acid to saturated fatty acids.

3. The diet contains familiar foods without omitting any food group.

Full interpretation of these figures and facts will come with more research. For now, the weight of evidence of dietary change for the average American and other peoples for whom coronary heart disease poses a serious threat shows the beneficial effects of dietary shift in favor of a slightly higher amount of polyunsaturates in fatty acids, but do not eliminate all the saturated fats from the diet. It may be this dietary shift should be made very early in life, for it could mean maximum benefit in a longer life with the vascular system showing less damage with increasing years.

By definition, three fatty acids plus one glycerol compose all fats. The stomach and, more specifically, the small intestine digest these fats into smaller components by means of specific enzymes. Some foods have small amounts of mono- and diglycerides added; the label declares such. These additions give a soft spreadability to certain fats and also furnish a greater range in temperature tolerance from a warm room to refrigeration. They are merely partially digested fats that are acceptable to the digestive tract along with other fats. As these digested products pass through the intestinal wall, they form again into simple fats, which the lymph picks up and carries to the blood. Although fat serves primarily as an energy food, it also provides support, insulation, and contouring of the "well-engineered" curves of the body.

## Proteins and the Amino Acids

Proteins received their name from the Greek and mean "to take first place." As nutrients, they not only furnish energy but actively build living nitrogenous tissue. The nitrogen of proteins makes them differ from the carbohydrates and fats, and because proteins, first of all, build body protoplasm, their position as "first" is seldom challenged.

*Amino acids* make up proteins and constitute the very building blocks of the living cell. Twenty-two amino acids occur both in foods and in body proteins, and although no food protein exactly resembles body proteins, food does furnish all the amino acids from which the body selects those needed to make each of its own many specific protein substances. Like the units of carbohydrates and fats, protein units are put together in food—the units being amino acids. Removal of water between each two units forms a large protein molecule containing hundreds of amino acids. During digestion, highly specialized enzymes in the stomach and intestine split the protein molecule with water at the junctions of amino acids until they are the size and nature the blood can absorb.

Given enough nitrogen-containing foods as well as sufficient total food, the body constructs some of the amino acids lacking from the food but required by the tissues. Adults, however, require eight essential amino acids. This term indicates that the body must obtain them structurally complete directly from food. These amino acids are: isoleucine, leucine, lysine, methionine, phenylalanine, threonine, tryptophan, valine, arginine, and histidine. The last two are needed in addition for infants and children.

A food containing amino acids in proportions and amounts needed by the body is considered a *complete* protein, or a protein of *high biologic value*. Examples of such proteins are milk, milk products, eggs, meat, fish, and poultry.

When a food lacks or has too little of one or more of the essential amino acids, it cannot of itself fully meet the needs of the tissues. Because such foods can only partially fill the protein needs, they are called *incomplete* proteins, or proteins of *low biologic value*. The legumes have notably low amounts of methionine, and the cereals little lysine. Besides being low in lysine, rice has little threonine; cornmeal and corn cereals are low in both tryptophan and lysine.

Complete protein foods, however, can effectively supplement the incomplete. Also a surprisingly good amount of supplementation results by serving two unlike, incomplete proteins together. Some admirable food habits have aided the human race in survival: the combination of milk with cereal, the eating of corn and beans together, or the use of rice with beans. Soybeans, because of their high protein content, are important legumes, and their products function very closely to a protein of high biologic value. One important consideration in supplementation is that foods furnishing different missing amino acids must be absorbed into the bloodstream at nearly the same time, for the cells that do the tissue building must have all their materials at the time they are needed. If the building is detained for long because of lacking materials, the whole project is scrapped, thus tending toward stunted growth and other signs of malnutrition. Many peoples have good and vital food habits. Never disturb cultural

Table 4    Protein From Some Common Food Sources

| Food | Amount | Protein gms. |
|---|---|---|
| Milk, fluid, whole | 1 cup (8 oz.) | 9 |
| 2% fat | 1 cup | 9 |
| nonfat | 1 cup | 9 |
| evaporated, unsweetened, undiluted | ½ cup | 9 |
| dry, nonfat, instant | ¼ cup | 8 |
| Buttermilk, cultured | 1 cup | 9 |
| Cheese, Cheddar or American | 1-inch cube | 4 |
| Cheese foods, Cheddar | 1 oz. | 6 |
| Cottage cheese, creamed | ¼ cup | 8 |
| uncreamed | ¼ cup | 10 |
| Cream cheese | 1 oz. | 2 |
| Ice cream, plain | ½ cup | 3 |
| Ice milk | ½ cup | 4 |
| Yogurt | 1 cup | 8 |
| Egg | 1 | 6 |
| Beans, mature, cooked, common varieties | 1 cup | 15 |
| Peas, split, dry, cooked | ½ cup | 10 |
| Peanut butter | 1 tbsp. | 4 |
| Almonds, shelled | 1 oz. | 5 |
| Cashew nuts | 1 oz. | 5 |
| Coconut, fresh, shredded | ¼ cup | 1 |
| Peanuts | 1 oz. | 8 |
| Pecan halves | ¼ cup | 3 |
| Walnuts, English, halves | ¼ cup | 4 |
| Breads, various kinds, griddle cakes | 1 slice or serving | 2 |
| Cereals, ready-to-eat | 1-oz. serving | 1-3 |
| Cereals, cooked | 1 cup | 3-5 |
| Wheat germ | 1 tbsp. | 1 |
| Fruits and vegetables, most varieties | 1 serving | 1-3 |
| Gluten, wheat, prepared | 1 serving | approx. 7 |
| Nut "meat," dark, solid | ½-inch slice | approx. 15 |
| Nut "meat," light, solid | ½-inch slice | approx. 9 |
| Soy vegetable protein: | | |
| chicken, beef, and ham styles | 3 oz. | 18 |
| Meat equivalents for comparison: | | |
| chicken, boneless | 3 oz. | 18 |
| beef, steak | 3 oz. | 20-24 |
| ham | 3 oz. | 18 |

mores in food unless better ones are both available and acceptable to the peoples involved.

Pages 178 and 179 give the recommended daily allowances of protein for sex, age, and condition as listed by the Food and Nutrition Board of the National Research Council. Food composition tables, such as Home and Garden Bulletin No. 72, help calculate the intake of protein as well as other nutrients, and serve as a valuable reference. However, for proper everyday use, the Four Food Groups lead all members of the family to the inclusion of foods that fill the need for protein both in quantity and quality. Selections from the food groups calculated on page 25 provide 57 grams of protein. This amount of protein is easily obtained by giving proper thought to the Four Food Groups in meal planning. Eating more or less total food makes it possible for each member of the family to have the amount of protein he needs. When additional food is added on page 26 to include sufficient calories, the total amount of protein is 69 grams.

Table 4 gives the common food sources of protein for convenient reference.

Digestion of proteins begins in the stomach and ends in the intestinal tract. Protein-splitting enzymes are highly specific in their work of preparing the amino acid building blocks for passage through the intestinal barrier and into the bloodstream. From this rapidly moving transport system, the cells pick up what they need to produce any enzymes, hormones, antibodies, or other protein structures that have a specific, vital function. The work of the cells is simple if the materials are on hand, but substitutions are difficult to make, often unsatisfactory, and possibly entirely unusable.

After the cells select what amino acids they need, the unused ones plus those replaced by new material return to the liver, which sheers off the nitrogen portion of the amino acids and changes it to urea. The blood takes this end product of metabolism to the kidneys, which promptly eliminate the excess urea in the urine. Urea is the largest solid excretory product dissolved in the urine, although small amounts of other nitrogen products are also excreted. For instance, the body excretes creatinine in proportion to the amount of active nitrogen tissue living in the body from day to day.

The Recommended Daily Allowances state the amount of protein needed each day; the Four Food Groups plan translates this requirement into terms of everyday food. Thus the body functions efficiently, for it has what it requires when needed without the possibility of under- or over-protein nutrition.

**Energy Metabolism**

Carbohydrates, fats, and proteins are used to build, but eventually burn to the extent of four calories per gram for carbohydrates and proteins, and nine calories per gram for fat. They add up to the number of large calories the body can use for energy metabolism. The body is in energy balance when the calories eaten equal the calories expended in work or growth. Too few calories lead to weight loss; too many, to weight gain.

Chapter 4
# IN THE ASHES

Foods that supply energy are not composed purely of carbohydrate, fat, and protein. Nature combines the energy foods with many other nutrients. When the body oxidizes calorie foods for energy, it leaves ash materials, or those nutrients which remain essentially unchanged. These minerals exist in food as various forms of mineral salts. The most common mineral salt is sodium chloride, or table salt. Even though many minerals are needed for the nutritional processes of the body, they are retained in small amounts. Only 4 percent of the body's weight consists of mineral salts found in both the hard and soft tissues of the body as well as its fluids.

After burning foods in the laboratory, scientists can analyze the ash to determine the mineral composition of each food. Food composition tables give the amounts of various minerals found in foods. These minerals are packaged together in foods in such a way that it is usually necessary to account for but two—calcium and iron. You can achieve this security quite automatically by planning the diet according to the Four Food Groups, making it unnecessary to check on each nutrient.

In certain geographical areas the diet may lack some trace minerals, and two minerals, iodine and fluorine, should be provided in ways approved by public health authorities in those areas where the water or soil does not furnish them in the minute quantities needed by the body.

All foods of the Four Food Groups contribute toward the mineral requirements of the body. Some are major sources, some minor. Some foods that contribute a major amount of certain minerals may have little of others. Milk, a major source of calcium and phosphorus, contributes very little toward the iron requirement of the body. No single food eaten regularly provides a large portion of the iron requirement. Rather, a number of foods contribute small but worthwhile amounts of iron to make up the day's requirement. Cereals, fruit, and vegetables all add to the iron pool, but seldom could their contribution of calcium give sufficient of this mineral to assure good nutrition.

**Calcium**

When growth, pregnancy, or lactation makes no extra demands, two cups of milk daily will meet the calcium requirement. Other food groups contribute small amounts of calcium but not enough to complete the daily requirement.

Milk is one excellent source of calcium, and all forms of milk provide equally efficient amounts in a well-utilized form—fresh whole, low-fat, skim, dry, evaporated, buttermilk, or any of the other acid milks. Ice cream contributes calcium but is not a major source because desserts should be used in relatively small portions.

A large serving (at least one full cup) of such greens as collards, kale, turnip, and mustard greens provides about as much calcium as one cup of milk. Cabbage, broccoli, and cauliflower contribute lesser amounts of calcium but more than most other vegetables. Some vegetables have calcium in the oxalate salt form, thus rendering the mineral quite unavailable so that little or none is absorbed. Spinach, beet greens, chard, and New Zealand spinach do not have much available calcium. However, do not avoid these greens, for they contain other valuable nutrients. Milk can efficiently provide calcium along with other nutrients important in bone building and upkeep.

An occasional fruit or vegetable may be a good source of calcium, but the menu maker must ask the question fairly, "How much do I serve of this food and how often?" Provide vital nutrients from foods regularly eaten rather than rationalize an alternate that you might use only on occasion. A serving once a week of a green vegetable containing the equivalent calcium of one cup of milk would replace but one cup of milk once a week. The fact that an occasionally served food is a good source of calcium does not give license to omit milk from the diet.

Calcium, needed by the bones for their structure, is also vital for the moment-by-moment maintenance of life. Such vital functions as heartbeat and normal clotting of blood depend upon the correct amount of calcium in the blood. Since the bones act as an emergency source of calcium for vital uses, a dietary deficiency may go unrecognized for many years. Serious decalcification of bones may be the first symptom, discovered only after the weakened bones fracture.

Table 5 reveals the importance of milk and milk products as a source of calcium; it also shows other foods that contribute to the calcium needs of the body.

**Iron**

The study of iron as a nutrient presents many facets of interest. The entire body contains only one tenth of an ounce. Iron is present in every cell of the body, although the hemoglobin in the blood ties up approximately two thirds of it. Oxidation or use of the carbohydrates, fats, and proteins could not take place without an iron complex carrying oxygen to the cells, and iron within the cell receiving the vital oxygen.

Iron, unlike calcium and many other minerals, is not excreted readily when excessive amounts build up in the blood. To safeguard the possibility of iron toxicity, specialized proteins in the intestinal tract under normal conditions regulate the intake of iron in the blood. The amount of iron absorption can be more or less, depending upon the body's need at the time. On the average, the body absorbs only one tenth of the iron intake. As little as this is (about one to one and a half milligrams), it equals what the urinary excretion, sweat, and skin lose.

Reproduction adds greatly to the iron requirement, and al-

53

though menstrual iron loss varies greatly, on the average a daily intake of 5 to 10 mg. of iron in addition to the nonreproductive nutritional requirement for the mineral will replace the loss. Because pregnancy and lactation carry approximately an equal requirement for iron, the woman needs iron in addition to regular body metabolism from the onset of menstruation until the menopause.

Egg yolk, legumes, whole grains, and enriched flours, breads, and cereals regularly contribute iron. Dark green leafy vegetables, dried fruits, and dark molasses constitute especially good sources but in many diets are used so infrequently that they contribute only minor amounts.

Only when most of the calories of the day come from the foods of the Four Food Groups are the iron requirements met. In many diets a large portion of the calories comes from various sugars, refined starches, and separated fats as found in sweet rolls, potato chips, and candies. Such diets can scarcely contain enough iron to replace body losses and meet growth requirements. Especially is this true for women, children, and teenage girls.

Table 6 shows the iron distribution in many natural foods. By including a wide selection of foods you can meet the iron requirement.

### Iodine

Most areas have sufficient iodine in the soil, but "goiter regions" do occur in many parts of the world, leading to the common occurrence of serious deficiency symptoms. In these areas, public health measures must supply this vital mineral. When the body lacks the necessary trace amounts of iodine, it cannot maintain proper regulation of metabolism. This condition may lead to serious developmental retardation in prenatal life or to mental and physical decline in childhood and adult years.

The use of iodized salt in cooking and table use most satisfactorily supplies this mineral. When a physician advises a low sodium (salt) diet for indefinite periods of time, he should provide his patient with another source of the mineral.

### Fluorine

Some underground waters, as they pass over fluorine-containing rocks, dissolve traces of the mineral. When the proportion reaches 1.0 to 1.2 parts of fluorine to 1 million parts water, the mineral greatly aids in strong tooth formation and maintenance. Such teeth are highly resistant to caries.

Since much of the drinking water contains no fluorine, large communities in fluoride deficient areas now fluoridate the water supply. This inexpensive and safe method of lessening tooth decay is especially effective in prenatal development and the early years of childhood, and if no fluorine is available naturally or artificially in the water supply, the physician or dentist can supply this trace mineral by other means. Adults also profit nutritionally from the correct amount of fluorides, especially as it may lessen weakening of the bones in old age.

### Water

Because every nutrient is vital, it is without point to compare the nutrients in this respect. Water, however, carries all nutrients and end products of metabolism. Water composes two thirds of the body weight. In positive health, water is in balance inside and outside every living cell.

Many tend to shortchange the body of water; thus, in spite of the abundance and availability of water, the body must "make do" on an insufficient supply.

The body obtains water from food containing liquid, from drinks, and from oxidation of all foods. When the body burns food, it produces more than one cup of water. Take plenty of good water as water, liberally, and especially between meals. Adults should put water drinking into their dietary habits and should also make water readily available to little children so that they can form good water-drinking habits early in life.

Most minerals are readily available from the foods of the Four Food Groups. You can readily supply those that require special consideration by following the instructions of local public health authorities. Neither old nor young should overlook the water requirements of the body.

## Table 5    Calcium From Some Common Food Sources

| Food | Amount | Calcium mg. |
|---|---|---|
| **Milk** | | |
| Fluid, whole | 1 cup | 288 |
| Fluid, nonfat | 1 cup | 298 |
| Buttermilk, from skim milk | 1 cup | 298 |
| Evaporated, undiluted | 1 cup | 635 |
| Dry, nonfat, instant | 1 cup | 905 |
| **Cheese** | | |
| Cheddar or American | 1-inch cube | 128 |
| Cheese foods, Cheddar | 1 oz. | 162 |
| Cottage cheese | | |
|    Creamed | ½ cup | 106 |
|    Uncreamed | ½ cup | 101 |
| **Milk beverages and desserts** | | |
| Cocoa | 1 cup | 286 |
| Malted milk | 1 cup | 364 |
| Cornstarch pudding | 1 cup | 290 |
| Custard, baked | 1 cup | 278 |
| Ice cream, plain | ⅛ qt. (or ½ cup) | 87 |
| Ice milk | ½ cup | 146 |
| Yogurt | 1 cup | 295 |
| **Mature beans (legumes), nuts** | | |
| Almonds | ¼ cup | 83 |
| Beans, dry (common varieties), cooked | 1 cup | 74 |
| Brazil nuts | ¼ cup | 65 |
| **Vegetables** | | |
| Broccoli spears, cooked | 1 cup | 132 |
| Cabbage, cooked | 1 cup | 75 |
| Cabbage, pakchoi, cooked | | |
|    (nonheading, green leaf type) | 1 cup | 222 |
| Collards, cooked | 1 cup | 289 |
| Dandelion greens, cooked | 1 cup | 252 |
| Kale, cooked | 1 cup | 147 |
| Mustard greens, cooked | 1 cup | 193 |
| Spinach, cooked | 1 cup | 167 |
| Turnip greens, cooked | 1 cup | 267 |
| **Fruits** | | |
| Dates, dry, pitted, cut | ½ cup | 52 |
| Figs, 1½-inch diameter | 3 | 40 |
| Raisins, dried | ½ cup | 50 |

## Table 6    Iron From Some Common Food Sources

| Food | Amount | Iron mg. |
|---|---|---|
| **Egg** | 1 | 1.1 |
| **Meat, lean** | 3 oz. | (approx.) 3.0 |
| **Mature beans and peas (legumes), nuts** | | |
| Almonds, Brazil nuts, cashew nuts, walnuts | ¼ cup | (approx.) 1.5 |
| Beans, common varieties, cooked | 1 cup | 4.6 |
| Lentils, cooked | ½ cup | 7.5 |
| Peas, dry, cooked | 1 cup | 1.1 |
| **Vegetables** | | |
| Lima beans, immature, cooked, carrots, cauliflower, sweet corn | 1 cup | (approx.) 1.0 |
| Greens, cooked | 1 cup | (approx.) 2.5-4.0 |
| Peas, green, cooked | 1 cup | 2.9 |
| Sweet potato | 1 med. lg. | 1.0 |
| Tomato, cooked | 1 cup | 1.2 |
| **Fruits** | | |
| Apricots and peaches, dried, cooked | 1 cup | 5.1 |
| Berries, fresh | 1 cup | (approx.) 1.5 |
| Dates, dry, cut | ½ cup | 2.6 |
| Grape juice | 1 cup | 0.8 |
| Prunes, dried, "softened" | 4 medium | 1.1 |
| Prune juice, canned | 1 cup | 10.5 |
| Raisins, dried | ½ cup | 2.8 |
| Watermelon | Wedge 4" x 8" | 2.1 |
| **Grain Products** | | |
| Bread, enriched | 1 slice | (approx.) 0.6 |
| Flour and meal, whole or enriched, dry | ¼ cup | (approx.) 1.0 |
| Spaghetti and macaroni, enriched, dry | ⅓ cup | (approx.) 1.0 |
| Wheat germ | ¼ cup | 1.8 |
| **Syrup, dark** | 1 tbsp. | (approx.) 1.0 |
| **Sugar, brown** | 1 tbsp. | .5 |

Chapter 5

# EVERYBODY LOVES A VITAMIN

At the turn of this century the word *vitamin* did not exist. When Dr. Casimir Funk discovered that food contained minute substances that were not minerals or calorie nutrients but were vital to life, he considered them vital amines (proteins). In 1911 he named these substances "vitamines." Soon after this date it was demonstrated that different "vitamines" specifically prevented and cured certain diseases that had plagued the peoples of the world for centuries.

In the 1930's and 1940's these vital nutrients were rediscovered from the standpoint of their chemical composition and function. The name had lost its final "e" and was now "vitamin." By the time the vitamins no longer mystified, the wonder was, "How can all vitamins be classed under one name?" Chemically they differ greatly and run the gamut of many types of organic compounds. Few relate to proteins in any way.

Changing the name by dropping one vowel sufficed, for it indicated that vitamins were just "vitamins" and no longer closely associated with the proteins, and the public neither wanted nor needed any other classification. Everyone loved the vitamins. Everyone hoped that scientists would discover other vitamins—known or unknown—that would prevent other dreaded diseases. The vitamin pill charlatans moved in almost as fast as vitamins were synthesized commercially. The vitamin-conscious decades followed.

Today the study of vitamins still challenges, but now the concern is how the body uses these vitamins and how they relate to the use of the other nutrients. The earliest classification of vitamins still remains their chief organization: the fat-soluble and the water-soluble. This classification roughly tells where it can be found, how well it resists oxidation or destructive change, and, to some extent, whether or not the body stores it.

There are four recognized fat-soluble vitamins: A, D, E, and K. Eleven substances known as the B-complex vitamins and vitamin C constitute the water-soluble vitamins. Five B-complex vitamins form parts of coenzymes and render vital services to the metabolic processes essential to the utilization of the carbohydrates, fats, and proteins. These vitamins are thiamine, riboflavin, niacin, the pyridoxines, and pantothenic acid. Two of the B vitamins, $B_{12}$ and folic acid, are essential to the blood-making organs of the body. Four vitaminlike compounds require no special dietary concern as they are readily made from other available compounds, or synthesized by bacteria in the intestinal tract, or not proved essential in human nutrition. These four vitamins are choline, biotin, para-aminobenzoic acid, and inositol.

Vitamin C, known as ascorbic acid, is essential for a number of vital metabolic processes. This vitamin keeps the tissues of the body intact and, in ways different from the B vitamins, facilitates the oxidation and reduction processes of energy metabolism.

As with all the other nutrients, a well-chosen daily diet from the Four Food Groups liberally supplies the needed vitamins. Substituting foods from one group for another will not assure the diet of all the nutrients. Heeding the special instructions of the fruit and vegetable group (to include a green or yellow vegetable and a citrus fruit) assures vitamins A and C, because it is possible to choose fruits and vegetables with minimal amounts and bypass the better sources of both vitamins.

A brief review of the vitamins shows how specific food sources are included in order to compose a diet adequate for all the body's functions.

## The Fat-soluble Vitamins

Each of the fat-soluble vitamins exists in several nutritionally active forms, each with its own name and specific chemical structure. No one name would describe all its forms any more than would the name of a twin or a triplet refer to all of the group. Because of this, chemical names are not commonly used but rather a "tag name" of an initial indicating the whole related group.

*Vitamin A*

Foods of vegetable origin do not contain vitamin A. Rather, certain yellow pigments of the carotenes in some foods serve as precursors of vitamin A. The intestinal wall can convert four carotenes into vitamin A.

Preformed vitamin A occurs only in foods of animal origin, because animals convert carotenes capable of forming vitamin A and dissolve them in certain fat-containing tissues and animal products. Thus butterfat, egg yolk, and their products supply this vitamin, as well as certain animal tissues such as liver.

Although the body utilizes preformed vitamin A more efficiently than the carotenes, a well-constructed diet derives most of its vitamin A from carotene sources which the body utilizes approximately two thirds as efficiently as the preformed vitamin. The animal sources, if used alone, would produce a diet too high in fat, cholesterol, and other fat-related substances for wise food choices. Therefore, it is important to rely partially on the very green and deep yellow vegetables. One serving daily of a green or yellow vegetable with the other food inclusions of the Four Food Groups amply supplies this vitamin.

Understanding the natural abundance of vitamin A foods makes it difficult to believe that many diets lack vitamin A. But since so many people have not learned to like a wide variety of vegetables, they often shortchange vitamin A in their diet. Include a variety of vegetables in the diets of young children —giving them tiny amounts (even fractions of a teaspoonful) with well-liked foods when they are hungry and continuing often until they acquire an acceptance. It pleases any hostess to have everyone at the table enthusiastically receive the vegetables served.

Vitamin A is not easily destroyed, but choose fresh vegetables in prime condition. The vitamin can be lost through oxidation (exposure to air or overcooking), but properly prepared food retains it.

A severe loss of vitamin A (as well as all fat-soluble vitamins) occurs through the use of mineral oil as a laxative. Therefore, never use such a nutritionally dangerous practice as a home remedy. Mineral oil is not a food oil; it is not digested; it is not absorbed by the intestine. It does have some of the characteristics of a food oil; one is its ability to absorb fat-soluble substances, which it does not release but are lost in the intestinal excretions. A child, especially, when given mineral oil regularly can become severely deficient in fat-soluble vitamins.

Deficiency symptoms of the vitamins are legion, and this book cannot possibly describe in detail the effects of vitamin deficiency on the body. In general, vitamin A deficiency adversely affects many functions of the body and appears especially in poor hair and skin conditions and growth abnormalities. A deficiency of vitamin A also affects the health of all living tissues of body orifices by the loss of tissue ability to remain normally moist or lubricated. Also, the eye may lose its ability to adapt quickly from light to dark (night blindness). Serious and continued deficiency causes blindness due to the disease xerophthalmia (meaning "dry eyes").

The Four Food Groups used as a basis for meal planning assure plenty of vitamin A. It can be obtained preformed in milk, milk products, and eggs or in pre-vitamin form from the green and yellow vegetables. Green vegetables also contain the yellow pigment, but the darker green pigment, chlorophyll, masks it.

It is easy for individuals or whole families to slip into the habit of bypassing the very green or yellow vegetables, and especially is this so with teen-age boys. At the very time the health of the skin is paramount, unfortunately teen young people lose interest in the foods that best supply the vitamins needed by the skin for its complicated functions.

*Vitamin E*

A normal good diet including a liberal amount of whole grains supplies sufficient vitamin E, called the tocopherols. Wheat-germ oil provides a concentrated form of this vitamin.

Large amounts of polyunsaturated fats increase the requirement of this vitamin, and although the body requires linoleic acid (the essential polyunsaturated fatty acid), do not use it excessively. This fact points up the overruling principle of moderation in all matters relating to nutrition.

*Vitamin K*

The "koagulation vitamin," discovered by Henrik Dam, of Copenhagen, in 1935, is essential to normal blood clotting. Present in very small amounts in leafy vegetables, egg yolk, soybean oil, and liver, under correct conditions it is also synthesized in the intestinal tract.

Physicians prescribe vitamin K for some newborns and for certain abnormal conditions. In fact, the knowledge of this vitamin and its use in medical practice is extremely important in saving lives of individuals with certain types of hemorrhage.

Under normal conditions, there is sufficient vitamin K. Under certain abnormal conditions, it may be used but only with medical supervision, for an overdosage is toxic.

*Vitamin D*

Sufficient vitamin D prevents the bone disease rickets. This vitamin aids in the proper absorption and utilization of calcium and phosphorus in bone building and exists in two principal forms. One is preformed in certain animal fats (some fish livers, notably), and the other is the result of irradiation of ultraviolet light (certain wavelengths of sunlight) on some plant materials; both are effective.

The human being can make a vitamin D by exposure of the skin to sunlight. Since it is difficult to regulate the amount synthesized from a type of cholesterol in the skin, the amount from this source may or may not suffice—depending on climatic conditions, personal habits of living, and the amount of skin pigmentation.

It is most practical to give babies, young children, and pregnant and lactating mothers a vitamin D source as prescribed by a physician. If necessary, he can also prescribe for older children. Adults have no specific requirement for this vitamin, but dairy and egg fats assure a small intake.

Severe toxicity may result from overdoses of vitamin D. Always follow instructions exactly in giving vitamin D, and use only the vitamin D supplements prescribed by the physician. He should know, for instance, whether or not you use vitamin D fortified milk and whether or not the child has regular exposure to the sun. Strictly avoid sunburning, for it damages the skin and provides no nutritional advantage.

**The Water-soluble Vitamins**

Vitamin C and the various B vitamins are water-soluble. As a rule vitamins in this group are easily lost in one or more ways. First of all, because a water media carries them, they can be lost when cooking water is not utilized. Larger food pieces and a short cooking time lessen inevitable loss of these vulnerable vitamins. Good cooks use enough water for rapid heat transfer but not enough to necessitate draining after cooking. Cooking with unneutralized soda causes excessive loss of water-soluble vitamins.

These vitamins are also water-soluble in body fluids, which means the body cannot store more than the saturation the tissues and fluids allow. Supply these vitamins daily, and guard against other types of losses.

The food manager who preserves vitamins guards all along the line of selection, storage, and preparation. Keeping foods cool, out of light, in fresh, prime condition, and cooking till just done form the best safeguards.

*Vitamin C*

It is easy to get enough vitamin C in pleasant ways. In a land of plenty, only ignorance, carelessness, or poverty could prevent an individual or family from having a daily abundance of this vitamin. Four ounces (one-half cup) of a citrus juice, a medium orange, or half a grapefruit will amply supply this vitamin. Also, tomatoes or tomato juice (one cup), fresh, leafy salads, fresh cabbage, and strawberries are good sources. Probably no other nutrient is packaged more deliciously.

The Four Food Groups specifically provide vitamin C. Neglecting its food sources in the daily diet is inexcusable. Many diets lack vitamin C because people expect a drink—any drink—to function as a real citrus juice.

Vitamin C (ascorbic acid) protects against scurvy, the dread disease of the early voyagers. Their diet of dried meat and hardtack with little other food contained none of this vitamin. Today's diet ideally has enough vitamin C not only to protect against disease but also to give all tissues of the body an abundance of the vitamin. When the diet includes sufficient vitamin C, the tissues are "saturated," or supplied with all they can use.

An abundance of vitamin C aids in keeping the cells intact, helps injured tissues heal more promptly, and helps the tissues resist infection more efficiently.

Adults should have 55 to 60 milligrams of vitamin C daily. Although citrus fruit or tomato provides a rule-of-thumb for dietary inclusion, a number of foods can substitute. Table 7 shows a comparison of servings of various vitamin C foods. The foods supply not only this vitamin but also other factors of nutritional importance. This fact illustrates the great value of getting nutrition from food, since the nutrients we know are packaged together so precisely and cleverly that we should plan our diets in terms of food groups rather than individual nutrients.

## The B Vitamins

Again, because nutrients come packaged together, we need consider only three members of the B vitamin group when calculating a diet. When thiamine, riboflavin, and niacin are accounted for in foods, the other B vitamins are present. The B

65

vitamins are also associated with proteins, which the Four Food Groups provide amply.

In general the B vitamins function similarly. They are essential to the effective utilization of the carbohydrates, fats, and proteins by acting mainly as portions of coenzymes that put the energy nutrients promptly through their many processes of oxidation and other changes. The final products of energy metabolism are carbon dioxide (excreted primarily by the lungs), water (excreted by the kidneys, skin, and lungs), and certain nitrogen end products (excreted by the kidneys). The B vitamins tucked into the diet by good food choice provide this efficient utilization of the absorbed simple sugars, fats, amino acids, and minerals.

Lack of the B vitamins has resulted in diseases that have scourged man historically. Beriberi, a disease that causes permanent nerve deterioration, is due to a lack of thiamine. People who existed mainly on polished, unenriched rice suffered from this disease. Less serious conditions caused by an insufficiency of this vitamin are by no means undamaging to the body. These symptoms appear as indigestion, lack of appetite, constipation, nervousness, and lack of mental alertness. When a combination of these symptoms appears in children, check carefully their thiamine intake.

A disease not known historically by name has been well known by its symptoms—ariboflavinosis. When riboflavin is lacking in the diet, a number of symptoms can appear: skin roughness around the nose and ears, a skin that appears shiny and pulled over the face called "sharkskin," persistent sore cracks at the angles of the mouth, and blood vessel changes in the eye. Salve relieves none of these symptoms. Only when each body cell receives the riboflavin needed to get on with the vital business of cell metabolism do the symptoms disappear.

Pellagra, once considered by most doctors an infectious disease, scourged certain Southern states, leaving in its path distress, suffering, and death. In the middle of the second decade of this century Dr. Joseph Goldberger, of the United States Department of Public Health, proved that pellagra resulted from dietary deficiency and that proteins of high biologic value could prevent the disease. Dr. Goldberger did not live to see the B vitamins identified, but thousands in his day benefited from his discovery.

Niacin quite specifically prevents and cures pellagra. Also, high biologic proteins, when taken in liberal quantities, have sufficient of the essential amino acid, tryptophan, which the body can convert to niacin. Dr. Goldberger recognized that the pellagrin's diet of refined cornmeal lacked meat and milk. The little protein in cornmeal has less of the essential amino acid tryptophan than most cereals.

Foods provide niacin as the preformed vitamin, or in the case of high biologic proteins as its precursor, tryptophan. Together, leafy green vegetables, whole or enriched cereals, milk, and eggs liberally provide niacin either in the preformed niacin or its precursor, tryptophan. In order to determine the niacin value of a diet, add to the total niacin the niacin produced from the tryptophan in the protein. To quickly estimate, divide the grams of protein in the diet by six, and add the resulting figure to the milligrams of niacin. To illustrate, the calculated choices from the Four Food Groups (page 25) provide 12.5 milligrams of niacin. The 69 grams of protein divided by 6 gives the figure of 11.5. This 11.5 added to 12.5 milligrams of niacin can be interpreted by this mathematical shortcut as a total of 24.0 milligram equivalents of niacin in the day's food choices.

Vitamin $B_{12}$ is not present in vegetable food except by action of specific microorganisms under controlled conditions. This vitamin, provided in the animal body, is in all flesh food and also in foods furnished by animals—milk, milk products, and eggs. Some food products have vitamin $B_{12}$ added. The addition of vitamin $B_{12}$ is especially desirable in foods to replace animal-produced foods, such as soy-formula foods used in place of milk. Good food selection easily furnishes the vitamin—for instance, two liberal servings of milk daily and three to four eggs a week.

Vitamin $B_{12}$ deficiency, or an inability to absorb the vitamin, causes a disease of the marrow of the long bones which make red blood cells. Nerve degeneration and a pernicious type of anemia

Table 7 Some Food Sources of Several Vitamins

| Food | Amount | Vitamin A (I.U.) | Thiamine mg. | Riboflavin mg. | Niacin mg. | Vitamin C (mg.) |
|---|---|---|---|---|---|---|
| **Milk and Milk Products** | | | | | | |
| Milk, whole | 1 cup | 350* | .08 | .42 | .1 | 2 |
| Cheese, Cheddar | 1 oz. | 350 | trace | .12 | trace | 0 |
| Cheese, cottage, creamed | ½ cup | 190 | .03 | .28 | .1 | 0 |
| Yogurt | 1 cup | 170 | .09 | .43 | .2 | 2 |
| **Eggs** | | | | | | |
| Eggs | 1 egg | 590 | .05 | .15 | trace | 0 |
| Yolk of egg | 1 yolk | 580 | .04 | .07 | trace | 0 |
| **Meat** | | | | | | |
| Beef, lean | 3 oz. | 20 | .08 | .20 | 5.1 | — |
| **Beans and Peas, mature (legumes), Nuts** | | | | | | |
| Almonds | ¼ cup | 0 | .08 | .33 | 1.2 | trace |
| Beans, dry, common varieties, cooked | 1 cup | trace | .13 | .10 | 1.5 | — |
| Peanut butter | 1 tbsp. | — | .02 | .02 | 2.4 | 0 |
| Peas, split, dry, cooked | 1 cup | 100 | .37 | .22 | 2.2 | — |
| **Vegetables** | | | | | | |
| Broccoli spears, cooked | 1 cup | 3,750 | .14 | .29 | 1.2 | 135 |
| Brussels sprouts, cooked | 1 cup | 680 | .10 | .18 | 1.1 | 113 |
| Cabbage, shredded, raw | 1 cup | 130 | .05 | .05 | .3 | 47 |
| Cabbage, cooked | 1 cup | 220 | .07 | .07 | .5 | 56 |
| Carrots, diced, cooked | 1 cup | 15,220 | .08 | .07 | .7 | 9 |
| Cauliflower, cooked | 1 cup | 70 | .11 | .10 | .7 | 66 |
| Greens, various varieties, cooked (spinach as an example) | 1 cup | 14,580 | .13 | .25 | 1.0 | 50 |

| Food | Amount | | | | | |
|---|---|---|---|---|---|---|
| Peas, green, cooked | 1 cup | 860 | .44 | .17 | 3.7 | 33 |
| Potatoes, cooked | 1 med. | trace | .13 | .05 | 2.0 | 22 |
| Squash, winter, cooked | 1 cup | 8,610 | .10 | .27 | 1.4 | 27 |
| Sweet potatoes, baked | 1 med. | 8,910 | .10 | .07 | .7 | 24 |
| Tomatoes, cooked | 1 cup | 2,180 | .13 | .07 | 1.7 | 40 |
| **Fruits** | | | | | | |
| Apricots, raw | 3 | 2,890 | .03 | .04 | .7 | 10 |
| Cantaloupe, medium | ½ melon | 6,540 | .08 | .06 | 1.2 | 63 |
| Dates, dry, pitted | 1 cup | 90 | .16 | .17 | 3.9 | 0 |
| Grapefruit, raw, medium, white | ½ fruit | 10 | .05 | .02 | .2 | 52 |
| pink or red | ½ fruit | 640 | .05 | .02 | .3 | 52 |
| Orange, raw | 1 med. | 310 | .16 | .06 | .6 | 70 |
| Strawberries, fresh | 1 cup | 90 | .04 | .10 | 1.0 | 88 |
| **Grain Products** | | | | | | |
| Bread, white, enriched | 3 slices | trace | .18 | .12 | 1.5 | trace |
| Bread, whole-wheat | 3 slices | trace | .18 | .09 | 2.1 | trace |
| Cornmeal, yellow, enriched | ¼ cup | 160 | .16 | .09 | 1.3 | 0 |
| Macaroni, cooked | 1 cup | 0 | .23 | .14 | 1.9 | 0 |
| Oatmeal or rolled oats, cooked | 1 cup | 0 | .19 | .05 | .3 | 0 |
| Rice, polished, enriched, cooked | 1 cup | 0 | .19 | .01 | 1.6 | 0 |
| Wheat, rolled, cooked | 1 cup | 0 | .17 | .06 | 2.1 | 0 |
| Wheat germ | ¼ cup | 0 | .34 | .12 | .7 | 0 |
| **Fats, Oils** | | | | | | |
| Butter | 1 tbsp. | 460 | --- | --- | --- | 0 |
| Margarine | 1 tbsp. | 460 | --- | --- | --- | 0 |
| **Miscellaneous Items** | | | | | | |
| Yeast, Brewer's, dry | 1 tbsp. | trace | 1.25 | .34 | 3.0 | trace |

*Bold figures indicate a highly significant vitamin contribution to the diet.

follow the depletion of this vitamin. Symptoms of the deficiency are much too severe and damaging to risk with careless or experimental self-imposed diets. Children are particularly and relatively quickly damaged by vitamin $B_{12}$ deficiencies.

In contrast to vitamin deficiencies, *hypervitaminosis* can occur. Overdose of certain vitamins damages the tissues and cell function, as do vitamin deficiencies. Overdose of vitamins severe enough to cause toxicity occurs with excessive accumulation of certain fat-soluble vitamins. Such conditions follow excessive overdoses of vitamins A and D either by accidental overdose or by the misapplied idea, "If a little is good, more is even better."

The nutrients—carbohydrates, fats, proteins, minerals, and vitamins—do not function in isolation but accomplish their work by a highly developed team approach. The Four Food Groups puzzle makes this "organization" work the best in providing adequate nutrition. A few well-chosen foods each day accomplishes the goal of excellent nutrition, and meanwhile the abundant variety of foods available from each puzzle piece not only makes eating an exciting adventure but helps the eater avoid nutritional pitfalls.

Add social graces and good fellowship to proper food selection and preparation, and you foster high morale. This aid to good living accomplishes a happy reaction toward life. At home, or at any substitute for the family table—lunch box or eating out —good food furnishing proper nutrition is requisite to life.

## SECTION II

## Food Fundamentals

Chapter 6
# FOOD PUZZLE APPLIED

To provide adequate nutrition for all members of the family, choose foods that fit together nutritionally, thus providing all nutrients. As critical as it is to provide the proteins, carbohydrates and fats, the many minerals, and all the vitamins, you can simplify this task by choosing the necessary amounts from the food puzzle and by interlocking them in one day's meals.

Examination of each piece of the Four Food Groups puzzle brings to light the classification and use of each food. Economical purchasing and wise preparation aid in providing the full nutritive value from each.

### Fruit and Vegetable Group

Colorful, mouth-watering fruits and vegetables add zest and delectability to daily meals. In this group lies the possibility of color to tempt the weary appetite, texture to please the dulled senses, aroma to stimulate gastric secretion, and an almost complete gamut of flavor. These foods add bulk to the diet without overloading calories. You can enjoy most fruits and vegetables as they are—delicious packages of vitamins, minerals, sugars, acids, and aromas.

Fruits and vegetables should appear fresh and in good condition without any signs of spoilage when purchased. When choosing fruit such as citrus and pineapple, weight for size is important because heavy ones hold more juice. Since fresh cabbage and head lettuce dehydrate with age, you can determine their quality by weight also—the heavier, solid heads yield more servings. Soft spots, brown leaves, bruises, or deterioration around the stem or blossom end indicate poor quality. Seconds, as they are often called, can be purchased to advantage if the buyer has a specific purpose in mind to utilize them promptly, and if the price is reduced in proportion to the quality. Clean vegetables before refrigeration—preferably put them in plastic bags or in tight crispers as soon as possible. Curtailing purchasing and storage losses reduces price per serving.

During off-seasons, canned, frozen, and dried products often provide good buys and lend variety. Many ask, "Do canned and frozen fruits and vegetables have as many nutrients as fresh?" Modern processing procedures and jet-age transportation have helped make canned and frozen products very comparable in nutritive value to fresh products.

When purchasing, let the price per serving determine value. In comparing fresh, frozen, and canned fruits and vegetables, the waste in preparation of the fresh product and the liquid on the canned product prohibit an ounce or pound comparison. For example, two pounds of fresh peas in the pod equal one pound of frozen peas. The number of servings in a can is based on the drained contents. If a can of product and a package of frozen product yield the same number of servings, then compare prices. Dried fruits, seemingly high in price per pound, increase in volume with soaking and cooking, thus reducing cost per serving. When comparing prices, always ask, "How many servings will I get from this pound, can, or package?"

Both price and use should help determine the selection. The purpose intended will determine the quality or type of product to buy. For instance, fruit to be served whole and in its natural state should be more perfect than fruit cut up in salads or used in cooking. If inexpensive sliced peaches, small halves, and beautiful large halves in heavy syrup are available, the use makes a great difference when deciding which to buy. For arranged salads you may want to choose the large halves, particularly if one half makes an attractive serving where two of the less expensive halves would be needed. Obviously, you would choose the slices for a cobbler in which you cut them up anyway.

Fruits and vegetables at their best need little preparation. A good washing, perhaps scrubbing, removes germs, dust, and sprays. Pare and trim vegetables as little as possible, using a vegetable peeler to avoid excess waste and conserve nutrients located directly under the skin. Some you can prepare without peeling.

Cooking adds variety, and what a variety of possibilities exist, especially for vegetables! All too often vegetables are boiled and buttered day after day, ignoring such possibilities as baking, roasting, frying, or combining various vegetables. Cooking not only increases variety in preparation, it hydrolyzes plant starch and makes it more digestible. Cooking also destroys microorganisms and stops enzyme action, slowing down spoilage.

If you do not utilize proper means of preparation, the fruit and vegetables can lose their nutritive value. Skin or peeling provides a natural protective jacket which keeps nutrients in the food; hence, when you cook fruits and vegetables in the skins or in large pieces, they retain the most vitamins and minerals. Large pieces expose less surface area to the cooking water and air. However, if you can shorten the time of heating by greater surface area, cutting fruit and vegetables into small pieces is justified. Utilize the cooking water in soups, stews, or gravy; if stored for later use, seal the liquid, cool it immediately, and use it shortly. Never use soda to brighten green vegetables; it destroys B vitamins and oversoftens the vegetables. When cooking green vegetables, leave the lid off for the first minute of boiling, thus allowing the volatile acids to escape and preserving the green color. Add salt either first or last; however, it probably enhances flavor better when added first. If you desire margarine, add it at serving time.

Generally use only a little water and a tight cover when cooking, but here again circumstances may alter the rule. Strongly flavored vegetables may be more acceptable if dropped into a large amount of boiling water and cooked quickly, with the cover off for at least the first few minutes to allow the strong odor to escape. You can cook vegetables high in water content—such as cabbage, onion, summer squash, and broccoli—in a Teflon or heavy skillet with a small amount of oil to prevent sticking. Stir them until they shrink, then cover tightly and let them steam in their natural juices.

A short cooking period maintains flavor, texture, and nutritive value. This applies to all vegetables. So-called "waterless" cooking may require a longer cooking time and result in more nutrient loss than when vegetables are cooked quickly in a moderate amount of water. Bring water to a boil; add vegetables and salt; turn the heat down as soon as boiling starts, and continue cooking until the vegetables are tender but not mushy.

When cooking fruit, altering the time to add sugar produces different results. Fruit will maintain its shape if dropped into a boiling syrup and cooked gently. If you desire a sauce, cook the fruit first and then add sugar to the hot sauce, remembering that the fruit will taste sweeter when cold than while hot.

Use the fruit and vegetable puzzle piece to splash color and variety onto the menu by following proper purchasing and preparation techniques.

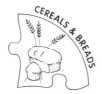

**Bread and Cereal Group**

Grains form man's chief means of subsistence; cereals and flours constitute as much as 80 percent of the diet in some countries. They play an important role in the low-cost diet because they store easily and because even in this country they cost the least. In the United States wheat is the most popular grain, being used for flours, cereals, and macaroni products. Use the common hard-wheat flours for bread baking and the all-purpose flour and soft-wheat flours for pastries and cake.

Barley, used for malt and interesting additions to soups and stews, is less popular. Small amounts of rye and buckwheat flours provide variety of flavor and texture in breadmaking. Rice may be the most versatile of the cereals, finding a natural spot in any meal of the day. Steamed rice as a breakfast cereal, rice pudding for dessert, and rice and vegetable casseroles reveal but a few of the possibilities. You can use oats, usually considered a breakfast dish, in breads, dessert toppings, and as an extender in protein dishes. Corn, often considered a vegetable, is a grain used for cornmeal, prepared cereal, cornstarch, and oil. Spaghetti, macaroni, and noodles are also in this group. Incorporating a variety of grains in the menu plan helps supply adequate vitamins and minerals. Many consider cooked cereals as breakfast foods, although their use need not be so limited.

When purchasing grain products, consider the nutritive value per serving as well as price per serving. Purchase at least half of the cereal products as whole grain and the remainder as enriched grain. Highly refined, unenriched cereal products have the least nutritive value. Many baked products and prepared mixes on the market use unenriched flour, so read labels carefully.

Pre-preparation of cereal foods often increases the price to consumers. In some cases they may cost too much, while some situations may justify the additional cost by saving time, storage space, and utilities. The homemaker should consider her time and facilities as expense whenever these are limited. Of the wide variety of convenience foods available in this group, sugar-coated breakfast cereals are the least desirable and most expensive. These cereals are highly refined, and, while they may have some vitamins added, they do not compare favorably to a whole-grain product.

Cooking raw cereal products increases the palatability, improves the appearance, and increases digestibility. Since the difference of degree and variety of preparation is so vast in the cereal group, rule-of-thumb instructions for cooking are not valid. Although the cooking directions on the package for hot cereals are the best guide, usually the less stirring, the better the results. To best cook regular rice, cover it with water, bring it to a boil, turn the heat down, and cook the required time without removing the cover or stirring. Enriched products have had some nutrients restored after milling, so do not wash them before cooking.

Bread predominates in this group. On the whole, use fewer baking powder products and more yeast breads. Baking powders are now balanced so that only a neutral salt, probably harmless in small amounts, remains, but quick breads are still not desirable for daily use. They also contain significantly higher amounts of fat than yeast breads.

The jigsaw piece depicting cereals and breads fits neatly into the food puzzle and offers a diverse supply of tastes and textures while contributing necessary nutrients to the daily meal plan.

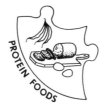

## Protein Group

All foods in the Four Food Groups contain some protein, but the amount of protein in one serving determines those to include in this group. The protein group includes meat, yellow cheese, cottage cheese, gluten from wheat, nuts, eggs, and legumes—dried peas, beans, and peanuts.

Each food in this group contains specific proteins, some complete and some incomplete which require supplementation within the meal. Wheat gluten and legumes (with the possible exception of soybeans) furnish incomplete proteins; they do not individually furnish all the essential amino acids necessary to make a complete protein which the body requires for building and repair. However, these vegetable proteins in combination can supplement each other, and are well supplemented when used with even small amounts of egg or dairy products, which do contain complete proteins. Many of the commercial canned and frozen protein foods available are formulated so that ingredients supplement each other.

Meat is a protein so commonly used that nutritionists often call the whole protein group "the meat group," but this does not bestow upon it top priority. In some countries, meat comprises only a small portion of the diet. Meat costs run high in terms of money and land required to produce it, and replacing meat with vegetable proteins may become necessary as populations explode and farmlands decrease. Meat analogues, as vegetable proteins are often called, produced from spun soy protein, wheat protein called gluten, or other food combinations make satisfactory entrées, supplying a good portion of the day's protein needs.

You can purchase legumes—which provide an inexpensive source of protein—raw, dried, or ready to eat. Make them edible by cooking them to soften the cellulose and facilitate the utilization of their protein. Make wheat gluten from high-gluten flour or purchase it ready to eat in a vast variety of sizes, shapes, and flavors. Meat analogues cost less per edible pound than meat. They have no fat or bone waste and do not shrink. These foods are tasty, nutritious, easy to prepare, and can replace meat in many recipes.

Eggs should be clean, without crack, and fresh or stored under quality conditions. Shell color or shape, unless extreme, does not affect the quality. Medium-size eggs usually provide the best buy for household use.

A few general characteristics apply to this group as a whole. All proteins coagulate or set when heated. Previous to heating they can be stretched. They form foams and can be denatured; that is, heating or additions of sugar or salt can change their characteristics. Too rapid heating toughens them.

Effective preparation of proteins involves consideration of the previously mentioned characteristics. Wash legumes—beans, peas, and lentils—and soak them so that they swell and absorb water. If you cannot soak them overnight, heat them to the boiling point in about three cups of water to one cup of legumes, remove from the heat, and soak for one hour before cooking. Boil or pressure-cook soaked legumes. Soybeans in particular require long cooking if pressure is not used.

Gluten, the main protein found in wheat, may be extracted and used to make entrées with meatlike texture and flavor. To make gluten, knead bread flour and water to a dough, cover with water, and allow to set a half hour or more. Then wash the starch out, kneading under water; change the water several times. As starch is removed, the water will be clearer with repeated changings and washings. A very elastic mass—the gluten—remains. Drop chunks or slices of gluten into boiling flavored broth; this causes them to swell promptly and then coagulate. Simmer the gluten slowly from this point for an hour to absorb both broth and flavor and to cook the protein without toughening it. If you desire a more tender product, leave in a small quantity of starch during the washing process to separate the gluten strands.

Since legume protein adequately supplements wheat protein, adding soy flour or mashed legumes to a gluten loaf is a good procedure. Small amounts of milk or eggs supplement cereal and legume protein. Nuts and brewers' yeast also supplement to some extent the protein of legumes. However, since nuts are very high in fat, use them only in small quantities. A guideline given in 1901 still applies to their use today. "One-tenth to one-sixth part of nuts would be sufficient, varied according to combinations."— Ellen G. White, *Counsels on Diet and Foods,* p. 365.

One egg provides six grams of complete protein. When preparing eggs, always gently but thoroughly cook them. Because eggs provide excellent growth mediums for bacteria, thick meringues, egg white beaten into cooked puddings, or raw eggs used in any fashion are not safe. Cook them at least five minutes. The Food and Drug Administration now requires pasteurization of all eggs and egg products sold outside the shell. Always cook eggs gently by simmering, not boiling. Hard-*boiled* egg is neither desirable nor necessary. In fact, *hard-boiling* of any food except when evaporating liquid is not a good cooking practice.

Dairy products such as ice cream and cheese may be included in the protein group if eaten in addition to the amount recommended in the milk group. Cottage cheese greatly adds variety, for it fits in so many places—salads, main dishes, even desserts. Macaroni and cottage cheese is only one delicious example of a cooked cottage cheese entrée.

This important puzzle piece appears complicated because of its many faceted components, but to summarize, always cook proteins gently. Soaking benefits legume and gluten proteins. Nuts supply a good protein, but use them sparingly because of high fat content. Combining proteins offers a desirable way to provide all essential amino acids.

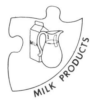

## Milk Group

Milk is a food, and as such definitely use it with the meal. Containing 13 percent solids, milk has less water than cabbage, berries, summer squash, and greens. Though it can be purchased in many forms according to its use, raw milk is not generally safe for human consumption. Homogenized, fortified milk is by far the most popular form. Nonfat milk and 2 percent milk fortified with vitamins A and D can satisfactorily replace homogenized milk, and contain less fat and fewer calories, yet equal amounts of vitamins and minerals. Use powdered skimmed milk —an inexpensive form of milk—in baking and cooking, or reconstitute and chill it for a very acceptable beverage. Powdered skimmed milk, when used exclusively, should be fortified with vitamins A and D.

Lactose, the sugar in milk, caramelizes when heated. This fact, coupled with carbon dioxide loss during heating, gives evaporated milk its distinctive flavor. Evaporated milk is excellent for cooking since it does not curdle as easily as fresh milk. Undiluted evaporated milk has a higher concentration of milk solids than fresh milk, and contains the nutrients of one full quart of fresh milk in each pint. If thoroughly chilled, it may be whipped to produce a topping or to take the place of whipped cream in salads and desserts. It supplies much less fat and more protein than does rich cream.

Commercial fortified soy beverages now available are particularly valuable for those allergic to milk. The same milk cookery principles apply when cooking with the soy product, since it is a protein food.

In choosing milk, consider cost and nutritive values. To analyze price, compare price and nutritive value of the equivalent of a quart of fresh milk.

Milk as a protein food requires special cooking techniques. Cook it gently in a double boiler or in a heavy kettle over low heat with frequent stirring to prevent sticking, scorching, and skin formation. The skin forming on the top and the part sticking to the bottom and sides of the pan are calcium caseinate, calcium, and protein. The foam that forms when reconstituting dry milk contains much protein; allow it to settle instead of discarding it.

Having examined the last piece of the puzzle, you may discover a favorite food or combination of foods missing. The Four Food Groups pattern does not have a dessert group, for desserts are not essential for growth or maintenance of good health. Persons accustomed to finishing a meal with something sweet may find that a piece of fruit will satisfy this desire. Include milk desserts in the milk group if you consider the actual amount of milk. Avoid the dessert that furnishes only calories, when too many have already been consumed, or that crowds out the day's Four Food Groups' requirements. Pies and cakes do have a place as a treat now and then, but consider them treats, not health foods. Including honey, whole wheat or soy flour, dates, or nuts will *not* turn a rich, sweet dessert into a health food you may eat freely.

Beverages play an important role in the diet. Fruit and vegetable juices are good, though the whole fruit has the advantage of the whole package rather than just the juice. Use unsweetened fruit juices more than the highly sweetened and artificially flavored fruit drinks. Chocolate and cocoa also have some nutritive value and are not habit forming. One problem with drinking large quantities of chocolate or cocoa is the amount of sugar that accompanies them. Chocolate contains much more fat than cocoa, which has had a portion of the cocoa butter removed. When used as beverages, consider them in the dessert class. Because of the high sugar content, also limit carbonated soft drinks in the well-managed diet. Hot cereal beverages and herb teas, free of caffeine, are enjoyable during cool weather or served at social occasions. Of the many beverages available, the essential Four Food Groups include only milk, fruit and vegetable juices. Choose these beverages for nutritional value; they require little preparation and contribute pleasantly and rewardingly to good nutrition.

Of all drinks, water quenches the thirst best. In drinking, as in eating, develop good habits. Water, although not listed in the Four Food Groups, is essential to positive health in quantities of at least six cups a day.

Many consider it unnecessary to bake bread except for an occasional quick bread, yet how good to come home to the fragrant aroma of baking bread. Nothing so establishes the reputation of a good cook as a fine loaf of well-baked bread.

Breadmaking is no longer a tedious, uncertain process. Fresh yeasts, well-illustrated cookbooks, electric mixers, and easily controlled ovens make success possible even for the beginner. The yeast plant requires food, warmth, and moisture for growth. In breadmaking, stir or crumble the yeast into warm water containing a small amount of sugar. This supplies the three factors needed for growth. After the plant permeates the bread mixture, its enzymes convert some of the starch of flour into the sugar the yeast needs for food, and it gives off carbon dioxide. The gluten of the flour stretches, holding in the gas formed and making the bread rise. When the bread is baking, it continues to rise for a few moments until it reaches a high enough temperature to kill the yeast and coagulate the gluten protein.

Yeast, food for the yeast, and gluten are the essentials in breadmaking. Add sugar, aside from the starter for the yeast growth, in large or small amounts as desired. Honey or molasses may be used for flavor instead of sugar, but the amount used will not appreciably add to the nutritive value. Add salt to give bread a desirable flavor. Salt also controls yeast growth; however, salt-free bread can be made satisfactorily. Since only wheat flour and rye flour have sufficient gluten to make yeast bread, use other cereals and flours only as supplements. To boost the nutritive value, substitute up to one cup of dry or cooked oatmeal, cornmeal, or other cereal or flour per loaf. When using soy flour, add only one-fourth cup per loaf. The fat used to make the bread more tender may be oil, margarine, or solid shortening.

Following a formula for breadmaking allows the baker to use the foods on hand and gives a variety of delicious breads. The following formula will make one loaf:

1 cake or package yeast (enough for up to four loaves)

1¼ cups water (fruit or tomato juice may be substituted for a taste treat)

1 to 2 tablespoons sugar, honey, or molasses

1 to 2 tablespoons fat

1 to 1½ teaspoons salt

3 to 3½ cups flour, at least 2 to 2½ cups of which is wheat

Any standard bread recipe explains the method of mixing. For a crisp crust as in French bread, brush the top of the bread with egg white diluted with one to two tablespoons of water. Brush the bread once before baking and once after it has baked twenty minutes.

Salads may be almost anything, served at almost any time. A salad can serve as the appetizer, the main course, an accompaniment to the main course, or the dessert. It may be raw, frozen, or canned fruit or vegetable. It may be largely or partly protein food or even cereal. It may be cold or hot. In spite of all this variability, salads usually have three parts: the greens and/or garnish, the body, and dressing.

The person who always uses head lettuce under the salad shows little imagination. Depending on the salad, leaf lettuce, deep green spinach leaves, curly endive, watercress, even celery leaves are attractive and tasty. The green base should be clean, crisp, dry, and fresh. It should never cover more than two thirds of the plate. A lettuce leaf split partway and folded over to make it into a cup is much more attractive than a flat, uninspired leaf. Since the garnish provides a spot for creative individuality, surely other possibilities than maraschino cherries, parsley, and paprika will suggest themselves, though these are very useful. A bit of olive or pimento, a sprig of watercress or mint, a wedge of apple or tomato, a slice of beet, are some of the endless possibilities. Any attractive color contrast, with a compatible flavor, adds spark to the salad. But a little goes a long way!

The main part of the salad should usually have no more than three or four ingredients, placed casually or mixed. A salad arrangement that shows evidence of excessive handling indicates poor workmanship. Salads arranged to represent animals, faces, and other realistic things are not in good taste except for children or some special occasion. Refrigerate the complete salad or separate ingredients until the last minute, if you plan to serve it cold.

Dressing and salad should complement each other. Why not add the dressing just before serving or pass it at the table? Macaroni, rice, some potato salads, and cooked vegetable salads may be marinated; that is, mix the dressing (usually French) with the salad ingredients far in advance of serving time—perhaps even the night before—so that flavors thoroughly blend. Refrigerate the marinating salad in a covered container.

In general, there are three types of dressings: French, mayonnaise, and cooked. French dressing, the simplest type, is made of one-third lemon juice, two-thirds oil, and seasonings such as a little sugar, salt, celery and onion salt, a dash of oregano, tomato purée, or whatever appeals. Put the ingredients into a small container with a tight cover and shake. Some prepared French dressings have gums or powders added as emulsifiers to prevent separation of oil and acid. In addition to the above ingredients, mayonnaise contains egg yolk or whole egg as an emulsifier. Cooked dressings have a starch base. Dressing used to its best advantage brings out and adds to the flavor, but does not drown the salad.

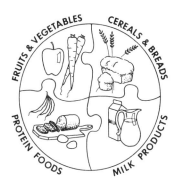

The food puzzle correctly put together presents a picture of complete nutrition for the body's needs. Time spent in careful purchasing allows everyone the correct amounts from the Four Food Groups puzzle on even a limited food budget. Proper storage prevents loss of quality and nutritive value. Skillful preparation of food assures that each needed nutrient is consumed every day so that the nutrition puzzle does not fail of completion.

Chapter 7
## CHEMIST IN THE KITCHEN


Similar to the way the matrix makes the preschool puzzle workable, so the chemist in the kitchen sets the foundation for acceptance or rejection of the food puzzle pieces. The complex foods, which provide nutrition for the body, have both chemical and physical properties that produce varied reactions during preparation and cooking processes. These reactions produce diverse results as cooking progresses.

As the laboratory chemist accurately measures and combines the chemicals for a desired reaction, so the chemist in the kitchen must follow directions exactly to achieve uniformly good results.

A standard cookbook gives recipes in a form easily read and followed. It lists the ingredients in order of use, with precise instructions, and gives size of servings and yield per recipe. The cookbook's size and shape should warrant easy storage. Pages which open flat and stay open for quick reference have their advantage. The recipes should use ingredients and utensils found in the average kitchen. Of what value is a recipe, no matter how delicious, which requires items one does not have on hand or expensive equipment one cannot afford? The gourmet cook may choose additional books or a collection of exotic recipes.

A good index saves much time, and the cookbook should include a glossary of terms used in food preparation. The experienced meal manager will find a Table of Weights and Measures, such as those in the *Pillsbury Family Cook Book*, helpful when cooking or when preparing a shopping list. A Table of Equivalents helps one determine how much raw food yields a specific measured amount. An example:

*Bread crumbs*   3 to 4 slices dry bread  = 1 cup dry crumbs
1 slice fresh bread    = ¾ cup soft crumbs

A Table of Substitutions can help when you are preparing a recipe and do not have a necessary ingredient. An example:

*Milk*    1 cup whole milk    1 cup reconstituted nonfat dry milk plus 2 teaspoons butter, margarine, or oil

If you want to experiment with vegetable protein, use the section on meat cookery as a guide, since vegetable protein foods can substitute for meat in many popular recipes. Additional desirable features in a cookbook include menu suggestions, guides to preparation, and illustrations. Pictures provide inspiration and ideas for serving. A good cookbook with good recipes is the laboratory manual for the kitchen chemist.

Careless *measuring* is probably the most common reason for recipe failure. Money spent for measuring equipment is wisely invested. Measuring spoons, graduated dry measuring cups (¼, ⅓, ½, 1 cup), a good metal spatula, and a glass or plastic cup with a rim above the one-cup line for liquid measure are recommended. An experienced cook with his personal recipes may obtain good results using nonstandardized methods of measuring, but even then the product might not turn out the same each time.

For accuracy, level measuring spoons and dry measuring cups with a spatula. Table-service spoons and teacups do not measure accurately. Spoon flour lightly into a cup without headspace and level off. Sifting before measuring gives greater accuracy and is recommended when the recipe designates sifted flour. The unsifted cup of flour contains about two tablespoons more flour than the sifted. This extra flour can cause dryness, peaking, and cracking in baked products.

Liquid-measuring cups need headspace above the one-cup mark to avoid spilling. For accuracy, read the amount in the cup at eye level with the cup on the counter. In recipes including one or more eggs use medium eggs. When a recipe with one egg is divided in half, beat the egg thoroughly and use half the total volume.

Measure solid fat by packing it into a dry measuring cup, leaving no air space, or measure it by water displacement. If, for instance, you need one-half cup of fat, fill a liquid measuring cup with cold water to the one-half-cup mark. Add shortening and push below the water until the water reaches the one-cup mark. Then pour off the water if not needed in the recipe. The shortening will slip out easily and completely.

Many factors other than the ingredients in the recipe also affect the finished product. *Manipulation or handling* may cause wide variation. Consider the beating of egg white, for example. First, a foam of large bubbles forms. Gradually the foam becomes finer and begins to stiffen. When the beater is lifted and a soft peak forms that turns over slightly, the greatest volume is reached. With continued beating, the peaks become stiff and dry, and the volume somewhat decreases. Decided overbeating produces little volume with white specks of congealed egg white. A recipe requiring one stage of beating will not produce an ideal product with another stage.

Stirring and kneading a flour mixture develop the gluten—desirable in breadmaking but undesirable in muffins and pastry. Overstirring causes tunnels in muffins and tough pastry. Insufficient kneading of dough produces poor quality bread. Adequate creaming of sugar and fat is necessary for acceptable butter cakes and cookies.

The *type and size of pan* are important. You cannot obtain a standard product when using an oversize or undersize pan. Using an oversize pan for whipping egg whites or cream results in poor volume. For range-top cooking, flat-bottom pans which completely cover the unit conduct the heat best. A pan which is too small for the burner wastes heat.

Glass, iron, or dark tin causes products to bake more quickly and burn more easily than a shiny tin or aluminum pan. A baking sheet with sides will cause cookies on the outer edge to burn before the ones in the center are baked. If you use such a pan, turn it over and use the bottom for baking. Bake most drop cookies on an ungreased cookie sheet and remove them from the sheet immediately when taken from the oven. Teflon-coated bake pans require no greasing and clean very easily.

*Environmental factors* affect recipe results. *Air,* although never a listed ingredient, is a factor to consider. Air conducts heat slowly, as in baking; it causes browning of fruits and vegetables. Covering to shut out the air or dipping in acid such as lemon or pineapple juice somewhat prevents browning. Oxygen in the air destroys vitamin C, whereas the acid and/or covering helps retain it. Air also doubles as a leavening agent—the only one in angel food cake. The egg whites hold the air bubbles, which expand when heated. First, the egg white stretches and then coagulates. Creaming the sugar and shortening also entraps some air. The grains of sugar are porous, and the shortening surrounding them shuts in the air. This helps make some baked products light.

A second environmental factor is *water.* Water conducts heat faster than air and prevents burning. It can help to prevent the darkening of peeled vegetables by shutting out the air. It often becomes an ingredient without adding flavor. Too much water, of course, reduces flavor and nutrients. Water softens, dissolves, and aids in mixing. Pure water boils at a constant temperature. Adding dissolvable substances changes the boiling point. Rapid boiling does not shorten cooking time; it only breaks up food, evaporates water, and often causes the food to burn. Once the water boils, turn down the heat to the temperature that will continue the cooking gently. One exception to this is in making jelly or candy, where rapid boiling brings about the desired result. Here it increases the concentration of dissolved substances as it boils the water away.

A third factor is *temperature.* Ingredients blend best but spoil quickly at room temperature. Heat destroys bacteria; freezing inactivates them; refrigerator temperatures slow down bacterial growth. Heat transfers more quickly through oil or shortening in frying than through water in boiling or air in baking.

Less fat is absorbed in deep-fat frying than in panfrying, if the fat is in good condition, held at the right temperature (a thermometer is essential for deep-fat frying if the fryer is not automatic), and pieces are fairly large. Fat in good condition has never smoked and is clear and odorless. Too-high temperatures cause smoking and chemical breakdown. Too-low temperatures allow the food to absorb too much fat and become soggy. Strain the fat after each use, as crumbs and pieces cause it to break down, developing harmful substances and causing greater absorption. Automatic electric frypans take the guess out of panfrying in a small amount of fat. Teflon-coated pans require no fat to prevent sticking.

When heat is applied to food, (1) water evaporates, causing loss of weight and greater concentration of the food; (2) protein coagulates or sets; (3) starch swells as it absorbs water; (4) fat melts; (5) cellulose softens; (6) colors and flavors change, a browning reaction may occur, and sugars caramelize; (7) some vitamins are lost; and (8) many complex chemical and physical interactions take place other than the more simple ones commonly recognized.

*Altitude*, fourthly, affects cooking processes. At a high altitude the boiling temperature lowers, and pressure cookers become very important to reach a high enough temperature to get foods done. Always adjust the pressure pan for altitude. You may have to alter recipes to include more strengthening ingredients, such as flour and eggs, and less weakening ingredients, such as baking powder, sugar, and fat. Depending on the altitude, increase liquid in baked products by one to four tablespoons per cup of liquid, due to more rapid evaporation in higher altitudes. Biscuits and muffins require less adjustment than cakes with a more delicate structure. Obtain recipes for baking at high altitudes and information regarding cooking from the agriculture stations of many high-altitude states. Cake mixes often include suggestions for baking at high altitudes.

*Acids and alkalies* may cause decided color and texture changes. Sometimes they are present in foods and water, or they

91

may be added. Examples of acids in food are ascorbic acid in lemon juice, acetic acid in vinegar, and citric acid in citrus fruit. Acids toughen fibers, turn greens brown, whiten whites, and brighten reds. If you flavor a vegetable with lemon juice, add it after cooking to prevent toughening.

Alkalies cause fibers to weaken and greens to remain bright but affect other colors unfavorably—reds turn blue or green, and whites turn yellow. Alkalies destroy vitamin C and the B vitamins, whereas acids protect them. The most common alkali used in cooking is soda. Never add soda to vegetables, because it destroys vitamins. Do not use in baking unless you completely neutralize it by an acid so that only a harmless alkaline residue remains. One cup of buttermilk or fully soured milk or one tablespoon of lemon juice neutralizes only one-half teaspoon of soda. Dark molasses may also be used—three-fourths cup to one-half teaspoon of soda. If the recipe calls for more soda than the acid in the recipe will neutralize, better use baking powder. One teaspoon of baking powder will replace one-fourth teaspoon soda, but less than this amount will usually suffice for leavening. One teaspoon of baking powder will leaven one cup of flour. Buy baking powder in small cans, stir and measure it carefully, and quickly cover the can after each use. Never use baking powder which has become lumpy.

Through everyday experiments, the kitchen chemist observes the many reactions resulting from chemical and physical properties of the foods in the Four Food Groups. Some reactions please; others are disastrous. Some of the food-puzzle pieces are delicate, others hardy. Accurate kitchen equipment and an increasing knowledge of food-preparation principles assure the chemist of desired results.

Chapter 8
# ARTIST AT WORK

In the artist's mind, a picture matures—combining color, balance, and form into a lovely creation. The food artist, understanding family needs for good nutrition and the principles of food preparation, sets to work. Colors, shapes, flavors, and textures of food furnish components for the masterpiece. The basic sketch for pleasing meals evolves from a well-thought-out and visualized menu, the table setting, and the surroundings; even the people partaking of the meal form the background.

### Mealtime—When and Where?

To successfully plan menus, first of all determine the time and place for the meal, for circumstances dictate mealtime. Where schedules remain flexible, two meals a day constitute an excellent plan for relatively inactive adults. When work or school schedules dictate three meals a day, it is ideal to serve the main meal at midday with a light meal in the evening. When the family is not together at noon, make the evening meal substantial enough to provide the remaining food needs of the day. A well-designed meal schedule discourages the current trend of frequent "mini-meals."

Plan a hearty first meal every day. Skipping breakfast or eating skimpy breakfasts robs many fine productive hours from the morning. Midmorning letdown, accompanied by the temptation to fortify oneself with the empty calories of sweet rolls or doughnuts, usually occurs about 10 A.M. Breakfastless individuals work below capacity until the noon meal takes effect in midafternoon. This trend has become so apparent and serious that some communities give children breakfast or at least orange juice and/or milk on arrival at school. Successful home artists strive to make breakfast so appealing that no one will want to miss it.

If the main meal must be at night, serve it as early as possible. Children usually arrive home from school hungry. A large meal at this time or soon after could solve the snack problem and the late evening meal problem. In many places school-lunch programs do a splendid job of providing adequate noonday meals. Carried lunches can definitely contribute to the daily nutritional needs if you use a variety of menus such as "A Month's Suggestions for Pack-It Lunches" on page 95 advocates. Drab, monotonous lunches disappear when the thoughtful artist takes over.

Home remains the most popular place to eat. What better memories of home can one carry with him than visions of the family gathering around the dining table and chattering about the day's activities? Must you always serve home meals in the kitchen or the dining room? No. More and more families like to eat on the patio, in the living room, or wherever they enjoy being together. Some meals you will eat away from home, at school, at work, or when traveling. Some you will eat out just for fun.

**Four Food Groups in Menus**

"What shall we have for supper?" leads to frustration if you leave the answer until a few minutes before mealtime. Planning ahead requires a few extra minutes, but it eventually saves both time and money. It saves time in shopping, preparation, and avoiding that "wonder-what-to-prepare" period. Institutions successfully use cycle menus; why not adapt such for home use? Repeat three-or-four-week cycle of menus over and over with changes for seasons, holidays, or other special occasions. Perhaps it seems that reusing the same menu means traveling in a rut, but the monotonous rut dredges even deeper with no planning. Getting the meal plan on paper enables the homemaker to see the job as a whole, and avoid dreary repetitions day after day

# A Month's Suggestions for Pack-It Lunches

| | Something Hearty | Something Crisp | Something Toothsome | Something Drinkable | Something to Surprise (optional) |
|---|---|---|---|---|---|
| **FIRST WEEK** | | | | | |
| Mon. | Peanut butter sandwich | Carrot strips | Applesauce | Potato soup (cream) | Dried fruit |
| Tues. | Nutmeat spread sandwich | Cucumber sticks | Orange, quartered | Milk | Date bar |
| Wed. | Egg sandwich | Celery sticks | Apple, quartered | Milk | Fruit candy |
| Thur. | Vegesteak sandwich | Assorted relishes | Fruit salad | Tomato juice | Oatmeal cookie |
| Fri. | Tomato and lettuce sandwich | Olives | Half banana | Milk | Bag of salted peanuts |
| **SECOND WEEK** | | | | | |
| Mon. | Soy cheese sandwich | Cucumber sticks | Apple, quartered | Tomato soup (cream) | Fruit whip |
| Tues. | Egg sandwich | Lettuce wedge | Jelled fruit salad | Milk | Peanut butter cookie |
| Wed. | Bean sandwich | Olives | Apricots (fresh or canned) | Fruit juice | Cup cake |
| Thur. | Tomato and lettuce sandwich | Stuffed celery | Half banana | Milk | Mixed nuts |
| Fri. | Peanut butter sandwich | Carrot sticks | Berries (fresh or frozen) | Milk | Pudding |
| **THIRD WEEK** | | | | | |
| Mon. | Vegetable weiner on bun | Nuts | Cherries (fresh or canned) | Milk | Dried fruit |
| Tues. | Tomato and lettuce sandwich | Olives | Orange, quartered | Milk | Stuffed prunes |
| Wed. | Cottage cheese | Crackers | Tomato, quartered | Vegetable soup | Molasses cookie |
| Thur. | Egg sandwich | Celery curls | Ripe pear | Milk | Fruit whip |
| Fri. | Savory garbanzo sandwich | Carrot sticks | Pineapple chunks | Milk | Dates |
| **FOURTH WEEK** | | | | | |
| Mon. | Hard-boiled egg (deviled) | Assorted relishes | Potato salad, crackers | Milk | Dried fruit |
| Tues. | Vegeburger on bun | Carrot strips | Peaches (fresh or canned) | Milk | Pudding |
| Wed. | Tomato and lettuce sandwich | Stuffed celery | Melon, peeled and sliced | Milk | Coconut cookie |
| Thur. | Peanut butter sandwich | Olives | Grapes | Fruit juice | Rice pudding |
| Fri. | Egg sandwich | Lettuce wedge | Half banana | Tomato soup (cream) | Dried fruit |

Reprinted from *Everyday Nutrition for Your Family*, p. 42. Seventh-day Adventist Dietetic Association, 1960.

without a menu. A cycle menu should never limit the home-maker, but provide security, while allowing freedom and flexibility.

The menu planner needs a place to work, preferably in the kitchen. Provide the needed tools—a file of favorite recipes, cook-books, pictures, new recipes to try, a sharp pencil, and eraser. To keep your file useful, weed out the recipes never used. Basic cookbooks contain lists of salads, desserts, main dishes, ways to prepare vegetables, and other menu suggestions.

Good nutrition requires top priority in menu planning, and including the Four Food Groups every day assures this. The four servings of fruit and vegetables will probably divide up into vegetables at the main meal, fruit at breakfast and supper or lunch. Oranges, grapefruit, or their juices served at breakfast will provide the daily serving of high vitamin C food. Tomatoes, strawberries, cantaloupes, raw or lightly cooked cabbage, broc-coli, or even new potatoes cooked without peeling may take the place of citrus fruit on occasion. One high vitamin C food in the day suffices. "Greens," broccoli, asparagus, carrots, sweet potatoes, squash, or pumpkin can serve as the deep-green or dark-yellow vegetable. One every other day from this group suf-fices. Consider one-half cup of a cooked fruit or vegetable an adult serving.

The four servings of cereal and bread may include a cereal at breakfast and one or more slices of toast. This group includes macaroni, spaghetti, noodles, and rice, but they should not fre-quently replace potatoes, as potatoes supply needed minerals. A cereal dish is a good idea for supper or lunch to ensure the four servings required.

Each meal needs a good source of protein. By providing sufficient amounts of cereals and milk throughout the day, two servings of foods high in protein will suffice—one at dinner, the other at breakfast or supper. Do not exempt cottage cheese, vegetable-protein food, legumes, or nuts from breakfast. Custom alone dictates that an egg constitutes the only protein food suit-able for breakfast. If you expect entrées to supply the protein needs of the meal, make certain they contain sufficient amounts of good-quality protein. If a serving will not provide two to three ounces of a protein food, a salad made from cottage cheese, or legumes, or a cooked vegetable such as peas or lima beans can supplement the entrée. Do not consider a dish made largely of macaroni or bread crumbs and seasoning a protein food.

The required amount of milk includes milk used in cooking. Three-fourths cup of ice cream or milk pudding supplies a half serving of milk. Milk gravies, soups, and creamed vegetables add their share. One-half cup of undiluted evaporated milk equals one cup of whole milk.

Good meal planning begins with the day's main meal. First of all, select the main dish or protein dish, then the vegetables, salad, and dessert if you plan to serve one. Three or four dishes per meal should suffice—a protein dish; a starchy dish such as potatoes, corn, macaroni, spaghetti, noodles, or rice; a cooked vegetable; and a salad or raw vegetable sticks. Casserole dishes, stews, or even salads including several vegetables and a good quantity of protein may furnish all the necessities for a fine one-dish meal with something raw and crisp as a side dish. Too much variety tempts one to overeat. The remaining meal or meals should include selections to round out the Four Food Groups and ensure good nutrition for the day. Breakfast need not follow a set pattern, but the average breakfast includes a fruit, cereal or egg, bread or toast, and milk. Supper or lunch may consist of a main dish such as a casserole, soup, a hearty sandwich cold or hot, or cereal; suitable fruit, bread, and beverage accompaniments. Page 98 gives some menu patterns for light and hearty meals.

Meals should satisfy the appetite and please the diners in addition to furnishing adequate nutrition. Adequate utilization of the simple food puzzle, provision of protein in every meal, and inclusion of some fats such as butter, margarine, or oil satisfy the body's needs and appetite. Fat and protein provide satiety because they digest more slowly and take more time to metabolize than starches and sugars.

# A Pattern for Meal Planning

|  | Light | Hearty |
|---|---|---|
| **Breakfast** | Fruit<br>Cereal and Milk<br>or<br>Protein (Egg or Other)<br>Bread and Butter | Fruits (2)<br>Cereal and Cream<br>Protein (Egg or Other)<br>Bread and Butter or Waffles,<br>   Pancakes, Doughnuts, etc.<br>Milk |
| **Dinner** | Protein Dish<br>Starchy Vegetable<br>   or Other<br>Cooked Vegetable<br>   (Green or Yellow)<br>Salad or Raw Vegetable<br>Milk or Other Beverage | Protein Dish<br>Starchy Vegetable<br>   (or Other Starchy Food,<br>   as Macaroni, etc.)<br>Two Cooked Vegetables<br>   (One Green or Yellow)<br>Salad<br>Bread and Butter<br>Dessert<br>Milk or Other Beverage |
| **Lunch or Supper** | Soup, Salad, or Cereal<br>Sandwich, Bread and<br>   Butter, or Crackers<br>Fruit<br>Milk | Soup and Crackers<br>Salad<br>Sandwich or Bread and Butter<br>Fruit<br>Milk |

Adapted from:
   Bogert, Briggs, and Calloway, *Nutrition and Physical Fitness,* 8th edition, pp. 494-496.

Pleasing the diner merits consideration. Family likes and dislikes will and should influence the menus. Teaching children to like a wide variety of food comprises an important part of fitting them for life, for good nutrition, and for social acceptability. A hostess and mother appreciates the guest and family who truly enjoy the food she prepares. However, allow every person to dislike a food or two. In writing menus do not entirely omit disliked foods, but serve them occasionally so that the family may learn to enjoy them. Buying large quantities of disliked foods wastes storage space and money, whereas small portions served in a variety of ways with well-liked foods give the unknown or disliked food its best chance for acceptance.

Aesthetic appeal dictates that each meal should contain variety in flavor, form, texture, and color. Foods of only one color or shape do not make an attractive meal. Serving corn, peas, and beans at the same meal or choosing four dishes each with a sauce or gravy does not appeal. Complement soft foods such as mashed potatoes, loaves, and soft vegetables with crispy and crunchy foods. Cooked vegetables can add texture if not overcooked. Use only one strong-flavored vegetable at a meal.

If you plan at least a week's menus at one time on a large sheet of paper, you will more easily visualize the meals and detect repetition of shape, color, and flavor. Avoid repeating a food on the same day unless in a very different form. Page 100, "Common Errors in Meal Planning and How to Correct Them," illustrates these suggestions.

Freezers provide service in taking care of leftovers and holding them at acceptable quality until they again become new to the eyes of the family. "Planned overs" remunerate menu makers. For example, leftover lentil roast from today becomes sliced sandwich filling later in the menu cycle. Or, you may utilize the remaining burger from one day's chili on a future day for patties. Checking the menu in advance ensures having items when needed. Even out peak loads for crowded days by preparing food ahead.

# Common Errors in Meal Planning and How to Correct Them

| Poor | Better |
|---|---|
| **(1) TOO MANY STARCHES** | |
| Noodles with Soya Chicken | Noodles with Soya Chicken |
| Mashed Potato | Spinach |
| Corn | Sliced Tomatoes |
| Bean Salad | Crisp Cookies |
| Rice Pudding | |
| | |
| **(2) TOO MUCH PROTEIN** | |
| Macaroni and Cheese | Baked Beans |
| Baked Beans | Mashed Potato |
| Broccoli with Almonds | Broccoli |
| Peanut Butter Stuffed Celery | Peanut Butter Stuffed Celery |
| Custard | Cake |
| | |
| **(3) LACKS VARIETY IN COLOR** | |
| Omelet | Vegetable Scallops with Tartar |
| Sweet Potato | Sauce |
| Squash | Sweet Potato |
| Carrot Salad | Asparagus |
| Sponge Cake | Cole Slaw |
| | Raspberry Sherbet |
| | |
| **(4) LACKS TEXTURE** | |
| Cheese Soufflé | Cheese Soufflé |
| Mashed Potato | Oven Browned Potatoes |
| Cauliflower | Green Beans |
| Molded Salad | Lettuce Wedges |
| Vanilla Pudding | Vanilla Pudding |
| | |
| **(5) TOO RICH AND REPETITION OF CHEESE** | |
| Nut Loaf | Gluten Loaf with Tomato Sauce |
| Potatoes au Gratin | Baked Potato |
| Fried Eggplant | Fried Eggplant |
| Frozen Fruit Salad | Tossed Green Salad |
| (mayonnaise, whipped cream) | Cheese Cake |
| Cheese Cake | |

Adapted from:
Bogert, Briggs, and Calloway, *Nutrition and Physical Fitness*, 8th edition, p. 492.

**Planning for Time and Abilities**

Making the menu coincide with time and abilities is important in menu planning. If you know that only a short time will be available at mealtime, utilize convenience foods, or prepare major items the day before. Often you can dovetail jobs, such as baking dessert for tomorrow while doing today's dishes. An automatic oven set in advance to produce the fragrant finished product as the family arrives makes a pleasant homecoming. Consider also equipment size and availability. If you have only one oven, this limits the number of items you can bake at one time. On the other hand, bake several dishes at a time rather than heat the oven just to bake potatoes. As a rule, a slight variation in temperature indicated on the recipe will not greatly affect the end product. The lowest temperature recommended for baking any of the items generally does quite well for the several dishes prepared for the meal. If one dish requires a longer baking time, start it baking before you put the second item in the oven. Time, experience, or physical strength may limit the abilities of the individual who will prepare the meals, and prepared or partially prepared foods may become a necessity. In a limited situation you can make specialties requiring extra time if you can prepare the remainder of the meal quickly and easily.

**Food Budget Facts**

The budget may require some juggling of the jigsaw, but planning ahead assists the juggling act. Limited money for food need not make meals dull, uninteresting, or inadequate. Neither does a liberal budget guarantee good nutrition, nor even pleasing and satisfying meals. Incorporate the economical principles of purchasing discussed in the chapter "Food Puzzle Applied." Then, supported by a shopping list compiled from the menus, you may avoid the pitfalls of impulse buying. Attractive food displays frequently form the financial downfall of the buyer without a plan. How much of the available income to spend for food is not easy to answer. The figure varies according to the family's size and set of values. Regardless of the amount spent, fulfilling the requirements of the Four Food Groups is the first prerequisite. Since this simple four-piece puzzle offers unlimited variety, altering the choices within each group can greatly reduce food costs.

Advertising alerts the food buyer of reduced prices on items in large supply or in season, and the wise shopper experiences substantial savings by taking advantage of advertised sales. Descriptive terms in newspaper advertisements, as well as food labels, indicate quality, size, and kind of pack. Price alone does not indicate a good food buy. In taking advantage of a special, do not allow impulse buying to lure you. Purchasing a large quantity of something the family dislikes or that will spoil quickly does not constitute a saving. Shopping when hungry may tempt the shopper to buy high-cost extras, such as potato chips, just because of an attractive display. Menus may be changed to take advantage of bargains and seasonal items. Almost everyone enjoys corn on the cob, tomatoes, and fresh peaches daily when they are in season. Buying an item just because it is reduced in price does not save money if you do not incorporate it into the menu.

All management requires flexibility. Circumstances necessitate adaptation, but planning gives security and a base from which to make the necessary changes. The homemaker well on the way to a successful picture of the food puzzle plans attractive menus from foods the family likes, thus supplying good nutrition within her budget of time, energy, and money.

## Meals for Special Occasions

A hostess need not feel that planning and preparing meals for guests suggest an overwhelming task. Once you master the practice of planning menus on paper, you can quickly write the menu for company meals. Why not tuck in the recipe box several special menus for immediate reference?

The special menus may include a buffet menu, a picnic menu, seasonal menus for planned dinner guests, and a menu or two you can quickly put together with foods from an emergency shelf.

When writing or choosing a menu for guests, decide first the type of service you will use. For a large group, a buffet is practical and pretty, and the wise hostess selects easily prepared recipes. Use a casserole, salad, and dessert that you can prepare in the morning or the day before. Make the cold beverage in advance and allow it to chill. Just before the meal, prepare the relishes while the casserole heats and vegetables cook. If you make the relishes earlier, cover them well and refrigerate. Spread the breads and pour the beverage just before you arrange the hot food on the buffet table. To generate smiles, serve a light dessert as a final touch.

At a picnic the hostess can enter into the fun more fully than in other types of entertaining. It also can serve as practice for more formal occasions. When planning the picnic menu, choose foods that require little preparation at the picnic site, or that keep well when prepared ahead. Remember during the picnic season the advice to be found in the chapter "Poison in the Pot."

Most families and guests look with approval at the picnic table when something new or unusual appears. New and appealing recipes from magazines, newspapers, and cookbooks provide fresh ideas.

For a spontaneous picnic, the children enjoy sandwiches as the main dish since they carry no lunches during the summer when outdoor meals are in vogue. A mixture of canned and fresh seasonal fruit in disposable cups, relishes, beverage, and dessert round out a carefree meal.

Meals including several families and eaten potluck style require planning to ensure a well-balanced menu. The hostess, keeping in mind the specialties of her friends, may tactfully suggest items for each one to bring. Families on a limited budget and working women with little food preparation time can enjoy potluck meals the year around.

For the more formal occasion, dinner guests anticipate an

appointment when they know a relaxed hostess awaits their arrival. The old saying "Practice makes perfect" applies in meal service, too. The unsure hostess can practice serving a formal menu to the family before serving guests. It is easier to invite just two or three guests to dinner at first.

Following the suggestions about preparing ahead, as for the buffet, the hostess will not give guests the impression of having overworked in preparing for them. By using a menu that includes two or three items which can bake together, she avoids last-minute crises.

Set the table before the final stages of meal preparation. When you invite guests for dinner after church, or for supper after a lecture or concert, set the table before leaving home. Then you can welcome your guests and spend but little time for last-minute touches and placing the hot food.

What about unexpected guests, however? Every hostess should realize that the meal is only a small part of entertaining. A longtime friend coming without notice will go away remembering a wonderful visit. When a stranger comes to church and you invite him for dinner, he remembers a friendly church. When a new family moves into town and is invited for dinner, they begin to feel they belong. Unexpected guests will soon forget the food served, but will long remember the hospitality extended.

Many hostesses keep an emergency shelf containing all the items required for menus planned for unexpected guests. These items might include ingredients for a quick, casual stroganoff, canned baked beans, or canned vegetables if you have no room in the freezer for any emergency items. Especially for weekends store in the refrigerator lettuce, cabbage, and tomatoes for a fresh salad. Dessert can be as simple as instant pudding topped with canned fruit and served with a cracker or cookie. Ice water suffices for a beverage if one is needed and you have nothing else on hand.

Do not avoid inviting guests to the home because you feel unable to please them. Although there are many rules for meal planning and proper service, today's society allows a hostess great flexibility in her own home. Advance planning and preparation free a hostess to enjoy the company of her friends while serving fancy meals on special occasions, and entertaining then becomes a pleasure.

A backward glance at the table before calling the family or guests should give real satisfaction to the home artist who has planned and executed her plan carefully.

## SECTION III

## Especially Tailored Tips

Chapter 9
# EXPECTING EXPANSION


Pregnancy especially requires the three-dimensional stacking of the Four Food Groups puzzle. At the moment of conception a new life begins, having already received all inherited tendencies. Therefore, parental responsibilities begin long before birth. "The physical conditions of the parents, their dispositions and appetites, their mental and moral tendencies, are, to a greater or less degree, reproduced in their children."—Ellen G. White, *The Ministry of Healing*, p. 371.

Parental eating patterns transfer to the life of the child. Mother's eating habits are particularly significant, for her nutritional status before the conception of the child directly affects both the body of the child and her own health during pregnancy.

The mother's body has a herculean task during childbearing. If a woman enters pregnancy in a well-nourished condition, mother and child encounter fewer difficulties. Diet alone will not determine the physical condition of the unborn, but it is one of the important factors. Expectant mothers who follow the Four Food Groups in planning well-balanced meals before and during pregnancy do have fewer complications.

The growing fetus draws from the mother's bloodstream the nutrients needed to mature and develop. In turn, the mother's body, even at this point, helps protect the little one from absorbing too much of any one nutrient. A lack of important nutrients such as protein, calcium, iron, and vitamin C affects both mother and unborn child, although poor prenatal nutrition more adversely affects the fetus than the mother. Toxemia, eclampsia, congenital defects, premature birth, or stillbirth are common hazards poorly nourished mothers must face.

"Have a second helping. You're eating for two now!" a well-meaning aunt may advise.

"Watch those scales!" demands the doctor. Who is right? Both. Expectant mothers must eat for two—one average-size adult and one tiny speck of life. The fetus gains weight slowly during the first half of pregnancy, and so should the mother. Fetal organs developing at this time demand adequate supplies of protein, vitamins, and minerals, and mother should choose foods high in protein, vitamins, and minerals and low in calories —such as raw vegetables, fruit, low-fat milk, and fruit juice.

Obstetricians advise strict weight control during pregnancy for three reasons: (1) excess weight adds more strain on leg and back muscles; (2) many complications of pregnancy and labor accompany overweight; and (3) generous stores of fat accumulated at this time are difficult to remove. At a time when women expect expansion anyway, some of the incentive for weight control is lost.

The pregnant woman should gauge her caloric intake to meet her specific needs according to height, weight, and activity. When the mother-to-be enters pregnancy in a good nutritional condition, at or near her ideal weight, she can expect to gain between sixteen and twenty-four pounds during pregnancy. This may be spaced as follows: less than five pounds during the first three months, five to eight pounds during the second trimester, and seven to ten pounds during the final trimester. She may use the rate of gain as a guide to caloric intake. Women entering pregnancy above their ideal weight should eliminate from their diet such foods as sugar, candy, jelly, jam, and other sweets, salad dressings, cream, gravy, fried foods, soft drinks, and rich desserts such as pie, cake, and doughnuts. If necessary, curb caloric intake further by using low-fat milk or nonfat milk, and unsweetened fruit, by reducing the amount of bread and potatoes eaten, and by minimizing the use of butter or margarine. Since artificially sweetened foods and beverages contain significant amounts of sodium, use them only with a doctor's recommendation. The chapter "Engineered Curves" gives more helpful hints for those who tend to gain weight too rapidly.

Servings recommended in the Four Food Groups for adult women adequately meet nutritional needs during the first three months of pregnancy. Since today's transportation makes foods available from all sections of the country, the consumer does not know if the food grew in iodine-rich soil, so a definite source of iodine, such as iodized salt, is needed. Daily eat whole-grain cereals, dark-green leafy and deep-yellow vegetables. During the second trimester, increase milk in the diet to three to four cups daily. You may substitute cottage cheese or American cheese for one cup of milk. As the baby grows and demands more energy and nutrients, increase the number of servings from all of the Four Food Groups.

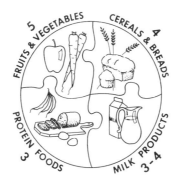

By the time mother has reached the last trimester of pregnancy, she should stack the Four Food Groups as follows:

Fruit and Vegetable Group ⸺⸺⸺⸺ 5 servings
    2 servings of which supply vitamin C
        (Citrus fruits, tomatoes, cabbage, strawberries, etc.)
    1 serving of which supplies vitamin A
        (A very dark green or yellow vegetable)
Cereal and Bread Group ⸺⸺⸺⸺⸺ 4 servings
Protein Group ⸺⸺⸺⸺⸺⸺⸺⸺ 3 servings
Milk Group ⸺⸺⸺⸺⸺⸺⸺⸺ 3-4 servings

Pregnancy during the teen years poses a greater nutritional problem and requires higher stacking of the Four Food Groups puzzle. Today teen-agers constitute more than one third of all women pregnant with their first child, yet girls in their teens have the least satisfactory diets of any age group. They seldom eat a well-balanced meal, but subsist on soft drinks and potato chips, or malts and French fries. Extremely weight conscious, they often go on crash diets, take diet pills, and exclude essential foods such as milk and bread because such are too "fattening." They rarely take time to eat a nourishing breakfast, but may snack on doughnuts or sweet rolls during midmorning hours. Since the teen-age body has not yet fully developed, eating patterns such as these can prove disastrous. Adding the stress of pregnancy to such a poorly nourished body increases the possibility of having complications such as toxemia, eclampsia, congenital defects, premature birth, or stillbirth.

Many young adults are anemic because of rapid growth during a time when their diet includes many carbohydrates and few essential vitamins and minerals. At the time a mother should supply iron and protein to build blood, tissue, and organs for the fetus, the storehouse is sadly depleted. Fetal needs take priority, so the unfortunate expectant teen-ager becomes even more anemic as her hemoglobin drops still lower. A hemoglobin level of fourteen to sixteen grams is important not only to supply fetal needs, but to cover the mother's blood loss during and after delivery. Women may lose up to two grams of hemoglobin within a few days after a normal delivery, hence a woman with a hemoglobin level of twelve grams can drop to the dangerously low bracket of ten grams following normal delivery. Therefore, expectant mothers, and particularly expectant teen-age mothers, should eat generous amounts of food high in iron and protein. Some iron-rich foods are egg yolk, legumes, whole grains, enriched cereals and bread, dark-green leafy vegetables, and dried fruit. Some foods high in protein are eggs, milk, cheese, legumes, meat, and prepared vegetable protein food.

Many obstetricians prescribe a multivitamin mineral capsule

for all expectant mothers. This may be advisable, for pregnancy is a time when their bodies have difficulty assimilating adequate amounts of all the vitamins and minerals, even when they eat sufficient vitamin- and mineral-rich foods. Women who have muscle cramps and aching legs may do well to consult their physician concerning lack of calcium even though they consume large amounts of fortified milk. Vegetarians do not always choose enough high-iron foods; thus, iron supplements may be advisable for them.

Since vitamin-mineral pills supplement, take them with the largest meal of the day, for the body absorbs these nutrients more efficiently in the presence of food. To ensure lasting potency, store vitamin-mineral pills in a dark, dry place in an airtight container.

Baby arrives—tiny, red, and a bit homely to everyone including his parents—and he is hungry. Without question, the most natural food and the best first food for him is his mother's milk. The first secretion from mother's breasts is colostrum, a clear, yellowish secretion rich in protein and vitamin A. Colostrum gets baby off to a good start because it imparts a temporary immunity to certain illnesses and may aid in the secretion of some of his own digestive enzymes. The mother who nurses her baby even a short while gives the newborn a nutritional advantage in life. When the mother nurses the child for a longer period, she greatly strengthens the benefits of nutrition and sense of well-being.

About the third or fourth day after delivery, the breasts of a nursing mother fill with milk, and she must not be alarmed at the watery, bluish appearance of breast milk in comparison with cow's milk. The quality of human milk varies little. The mother who desires to breast-feed her infant should keep three important factors in mind. First, after she has decided to nurse her baby despite a few discomforts and inconveniences, she must not worry about the quality or quantity of her milk. Tension and worry inhibit milk production. Ironically, the woman who is most concerned and apprehensive about her ability to breast-

113

feed is less likely to do so. Mothers who can provide only part of the baby's need for milk should feel satisfied that they have contributed significantly to the baby's welfare. Second, because fluids stimulate milk production, she should avoid dehydration by drinking at least one quart of milk plus two to three quarts of other fluids daily. Third, though difficult with a new baby in the house, she should take time to rest and relax, since it is essential to carefree nursing. Perhaps a spotless, organized house is not as important right now as a well-fed, comforted infant.

Human milk differs from cow's milk in several respects. It contains less calcium and protein, which a rapidly growing bovine may need in large quantities, but not a human infant, who develops more slowly. In baby's stomach the protein of human milk divides into smaller, softer curds, which better suit the digestive processes of the newborn child. Breast milk also better fills the child's need because it contains more of the special carbohydrate, lactose. In addition to supplying the child with the nutrients he needs in a form he can best utilize, breast-feeding gives the infant a special feeling of comfort and security. Breast-fed babies have less colic, fewer illnesses, and less constipation.

To the mother, breast-feeding has the advantages of being safe and sanitary without the work of formula sterilization or the possibility of error. Economically, it costs less than formulas. It is always the right temperature and requires no preparation time. A mother breast-feeding her infant feels a warm satisfaction in answering the need of the tiny, eager mouth with her own milk. When the mother leaves the hospital to return home, increased activity and anxiety may cause milk flow to temporarily dwindle, especially for the evening feeding, and mother may supplement breast milk with a bottle feeding after baby has completely emptied one or both breasts. The first few days at home should not discourage mother about her quantity of milk. If she refuses to worry or fret and supplements only when necessary, she and baby will soon work out a smooth schedule, satisfactory to both. If times of acute infection must interrupt breast-feeding, the mother can often return to nursing the child if she pumps the breast to stimulate continued milk flow.

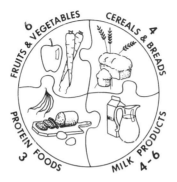

To provide the minimal nutrients needed, the mother who breast-feeds her child stacks the Four Food Groups as follows:

Vegetable and Fruit Group ........................... 6 servings
    3 servings of which supply vitamin C
        (Citrus fruits, tomatoes, cabbage, strawberries, etc.)
    1 serving of which supplies vitamin A
        (A very dark green or yellow vegetable)
Cereal and Bread Group ........................... 4 servings
Protein Group ........................................... 3 servings
Milk Group ........................................... 4-6 servings
    (Part of this may be taken in the form of cheese and
    other milk products)

Add servings from each group to meet the energy needs of the mother. Such a large quantity of food may be divided into four meals a day, or three meals and two regularly scheduled snacks. When baby is weaned, mother must remember to diminish her intake so that she will not gain unwanted pounds.

Not every mother can, or cares to, breast-feed her infant. Inability to produce enough milk to meet at least a regular portion of the child's needs, social stigma, the need to return to work, or chronic illness, such as tuberculosis, may require bottle feedings. Mothers of bottle-fed infants should not feel guilty.

The doctor will prescribe a formula for bottle feeding which will adequately meet the infant's nutritional needs. Today's market offers a wide spectrum of carefully prepared formulas from various sources and in several forms, such as powder, condensed liquid, ready-to-use liquid, and disposable nursers filled, sterilized, and ready for use. With ease of preparation, however, often comes an increase in cost. Many doctors prescribe evaporated, homogenized, or low-fat milk formulated for the individual baby's requirement.

Most babies love to be held. Whether feeding from the breast or bottle, always hold the infant; nothing can replace human contact. Aside from the need to be watched during feeding to prevent choking and coughing, babies thrive on the secure feeling of mother's touch and the warmth and comfort of her closeness. Holding the child also gives mother a good excuse to relax, prop up her tired feet, and enjoy God's gift of motherhood. But, most of all, babies need to associate happy, contented feelings with mealtime.

Chapter 10
## TODDLER TO TEEN

One of mother's first concerns upon arriving home with her tiny pink angel is feeding it. When? How much? What? The Four Food Groups does not give much assistance for this one short period.

A few years ago, doctors sent mother and newborn home on a very strict four-hour schedule, whether baby screamed with hunger after two and a half hours or wanted to sleep peacefully for five hours. Doctors were satisfied—babies were frustrated —and mothers were exhausted. More recently, physicians advise mothers to let baby establish his own schedule, which he will generally do within a few days after arriving home. Baby will often deviate as much as half an hour either side of a set feeding schedule, but do not feed him every time he cries; you soon learn to distinguish between the cry of hunger and the cry of other discomforts.

"How can I tell if my baby eats enough?" wonder many nursing mothers. The infant probably gets enough to eat if he seems satisfied after about fifteen minutes of eating, if he falls asleep after eating and sleeps for several hours, or if he shows satisfactory weight gain. At birth, baby needs from 800 to 1,200 calories a day. Human milk and most of the prepared formulas contain twenty calories per ounce, so a newborn baby should take from eighteen to twenty-five ounces a day.

The infant grows rapidly during his first year. Since each baby is an individual, his rate of development cannot be measured by a precise standard. The average baby doubles his birth weight by five months, and triples it by one year. We can under-

117

stand such a tremendous weight gain by putting it in terms of adult weight. If an adult gained at such a rate, a 125-pound person would weigh 250 pounds in five months and tip the scales at 375 pounds after twelve months. No wonder infant nutrition is so important!

"Hey! What's that lumpy stuff mom's stuck in my mouth? I'm going to gag!" Junior may react to his first solid food.

Twenty years have seen many controversial theories regarding when to start solid foods. A few years ago, cereals, fruit, and vegetables were not introduced until the child reached twelve to eighteen months; but now the pendulum has swung over to where mothers brag about the quantity of cereal their two-and-a-half-week-old consumes. After weighing the advantages and disadvantages, most nutritionists agree that a baby needs and accepts solids at about two and a half to three months of age. With breast-feeding you need not add supplemental foods as early. The development and appetite of a baby, rather than chronological age, should determine when you add solid foods.

Cereals are usually the first solid food given. Enriched cereals supplement baby's iron-poor milk diet. A normal full-term infant does not require earlier additions of iron, because at birth the child's liver reserves iron to tide him over the all-milk period of his life. Orange juice and pureed fruit and vegetables may follow soon after cereal, with hard-boiled egg yolks, custards, and cottage cheese added after six months. Baby should eat bland food with very little additional salt or sweetener. Adults may enjoy condiments and spices, but they should not use them for seasoning baby's food.

Many women do not realize that even infants need water. Acquaint baby with the taste of water during his first few months so that it will be a regular part of his diet now, and for the rest of his life. Older children may not care for water if they established their eating habits before mother regularly introduced water. Boil water and cool it to room temperature for the infant's bottle, and offer water in a cup several times a day to the toddler. Always offer the water without hurry and without concern; if the child refuses it, just offer it again a little later.

A baby accepts new foods best when he is hungry and not overly tired. They should be introduced one at a time in tiny amounts, accompanied by some of his favorite foods. The young baby is not adept at carrying solid food from the front to the back of the mouth. Therefore, place only half spoonfuls well back on the tongue with the baby semireclined, until he improves his swallowing skills. Give him several days to adjust to one new food before you add another. Do not force a baby to eat a food he does not care for; instead, an item he refuses should not appear on the menu again for a few days. If he still refuses the food, substitute a food equal in nutritional value and offer the rejected food again a month or so later. A baby will quickly sense others' dislike for food he eats.

Keep rich desserts and pastry to a minimum so that the child does not early acquire a taste for sweets to the exclusion of other foods. Feed baby foods varying in both taste and texture toward the end of the first year. The child accustomed to many kinds of food will less likely be a finicky eater.

Wean from the bottle to the cup during the latter part of the first year; at about five months, baby should discover how to drink from a cup. By nine months, offer a cup of milk instead of one feeding. Then gradually replace all breast or bottle feedings by the cup, although the morning and bedtime bottles may continue for some time. Nursing mothers discover that a gradual weaning, placing less and less demands on the mammary glands, slows the flow of milk and minimizes discomfort, and baby will rarely experience any physical discomfort or emotional trauma during a gradual transition to cow's milk from breast or formula feeding. When a healthy baby takes more than one bottle or nursing a day after a year or fifteen months, he may become anemic due to exclusion of solid foods containing essential vitamins and minerals.

Sometime during the second year, when a child can pick up objects between the thumb and index finger, he will try feeding himself, much to a tidy mother's dismay. For the next few months, temporarily abandon table manners as the child explores the texture of his food and develops his own dexterity. Although you need not tolerate playing with food, baby enjoys feeling his oatmeal and testing its possibilities. As he begins to master the spoons, mother may gently encourage a few social graces, keeping in mind that she should not meet the inevitable accidents with disapproval or scolding.

The second year, the child's growth rate slows, and he enters the "Terrible Two's." Suddenly, a normal, hearty eater picks at his food or even rejects entire meals. Parents must keep calm, for a healthy, active child *will* eat when he is hungry, since he can probably judge the amounts (but not kinds) of food he needs better than his parents. Since his growth rate has decreased, so has his appetite.

This period triggers many problem eaters. Junior refuses to eat—mother panics! She bribes him with toys and desserts—he whines. She threatens spankings and early bedtime—he clamps his lips and kicks his high chair. She tries "one bite for grandpa and one bite for teddy bear"—and he spits.

Mother thinks, "He'll get sick if he doesn't eat."

Junior thinks, "This is great! I'll try it again tomorrow." And so the long battle begins.

What should mother do? If she presents nourishing, attractive food in easy-to-handle forms at regular intervals with no appetite-dulling snacks between times, the healthy, active toddler will eat all he needs. If he refuses a meal, excuse him without a fuss, not to eat again until he is ready for a meal. The child given an unnecessary amount of parental supervision and vigilance usually develops into a problem eater. Orphanages and large families have very few picky eaters because they have no time for individual pampering.

Serve the variety of foods in the Four Food Groups in *small portions* to the toddler. The total daily intake recommended is as follows:

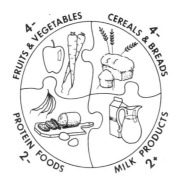

Fruit and Vegetable Group _____ 4 servings
  Include at least 4 ounces of orange juice or other vitamin-
    C-rich food.
  Portions of other foods may be 2-3 tablespoons.
  Include a dark-green or yellow vegetable daily.
Bread and Cereal Group _____ 4 servings
  Half slices of bread and 2-3 level tablespoon portions of
    cereal may count as servings for children.
Protein Group _____ 2 servings
  Include an egg 3 or 4 times a week.
  Give other high protein foods once or twice a day in 2-3
    tablespoon amounts.
Milk Group
  Three cups or more may be given if not displacing other
    foods. The child may take less or very small amounts
    of milk for short periods of time without harm.

Better serve small portions and then repeat as desired rather
than start with a discouragingly large portion of food. Follow the
rule, one tablespoon (standard measuring type) of food for each
year of age. The toddler may need five or six regularly scheduled
feedings a day rather than three large meals. He will more easily
eat and better tolerate soft foods, simply prepared. Avoid skins
and seeds of fruits, rich sauces, and fried foods.

**Preschool Children**

Preschoolers are delightful, busy creatures. Mother, who waited anxiously for baby to walk, now wishes he would occasionally stop running. The preschooler finds many new and wonderful things to explore—including food.

The preschooler usually prefers plain food—no gravies, sauces, spices, and very few mixtures. Preschool children generally prefer mild-flavored foods because of high sensitivity to taste; they find rich, sweet, or spicy foods strong and distasteful. They frequently prefer raw vegetables. The child's ability to chew should somewhat determine the texture of his food.

Capitalize upon chewing as a new venture to the young one with new teeth. The youngster will relish crispy carrots, crunchy zwieback, juicy apple or pear slices, and refreshing lettuce wedges. Finger foods rate high. A child may refuse certain foods because they are clumsy to manage at the end of a spoon, and not because of their taste. A large spear of broccoli may appear forbidding to small, chubby fingers, whereas he can easily pick up one or two small broccoli buds to explore. He may tire of eating cereal with a spoon, but he will thrill if it is thick and offered to him as finger-food balls.

Desire for food may be erratic for the preschooler, so an occasional "won't eat" phase should not cause undue concern. A healthy child eventually gets hungry and eats satisfactorily over a period of time. On the other hand, food jags frequent the preschool years. If Johnny decides he will exist on peanut butter sandwiches and celery sticks for a day or two, it is no disaster. Accept the food jags instead of blowing them out of proportion, and he will abandon them in due time. Parents, instead of putting too much emphasis on eating, should establish mealtime as a happy, relaxed family occasion.

A child tends to dawdle at this age. Fortunately, he does not have the adult sense of time and does not feel rushed. Urging him to "hurry" may spoil his pleasure in life and in eating. Why not let the child begin his meal before the rest of the family sits down so that you need not rush him? A child served small portions, or allowed to serve himself, may do a better job of eating everything on his plate. Making a "clean plate" a familiar rule may lead to a habit of overeating which can carry over into later life and lead to overweight. Many mothers wonder whether to allow a child who leaves food on his plate to eat dessert. If dessert is an occasional treat, as it should be, the problem solves itself. As a rule, a fair consumption of food served on the plate justifies at least a small serving of dessert eaten with the rest of the family. Far better to set a good example in eating for Junior to follow than to nag.

Active children may become overtired and, although excessively hungry, cannot eat properly. Proper rest, plus regular snacks in midmorning and/or midafternoon may correct this. Serve snacks light enough not to spoil the appetite for the next meal and make them contribute to the child's nutritional need. Such snack foods may be fruit juice, milk, dry cereal, plain crackers, or bread.

When children snack on candy, soft drinks, potato chips, and empty calorie foods virtually all day and are big enough to help themselves, many parents wail, "I haven't time to watch them every minute. I just cannot do anything about it." The answer is simple. Never store candy, chips, soft drinks, etc., because they tempt children and adults alike. Instead, a wise mother furnishes nutritious snack possibilities, such as carrot and celery strips, fresh fruits, whole-grain breads, and unsweetened cereals.

Chubby, dimpled five-year-olds delight parents and photographers but worry nutritionists. Most normal four-to-five-year-olds are thin and gangly. The cute, plump five-year-old often matures into the obese adult who battles overweight for a lifetime. This amplifies the significance of utilizing the Four Food Groups puzzle, emphasizing more fruit and vegetables and less sweets, desserts, empty calorie snacks, and excess starchy foods.

**School Age**

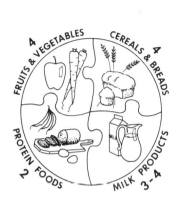

Play activities easily divert eager, happy-go-lucky grade school youngsters from eating. Without vigilant mothers, "Little Leaguers" grab a slice of bread and peanut butter and race off to the ball field. If schools did not require students to remain in their seats or in the cafeteria for at least fifteen minutes during noon hour, most children would skip lunch in favor of play.

In general, the school-age child copies the eating habits of those about him. If teacher has chocolate-marshmallow cookies every day for lunch, then "Little Miss" must eat chocolate-marshmallow cookies every day for lunch. The child compares home eating habits with the eating habits of his peers, thus discovering that the world encompasses much more than his small family circle. Group influence is important, and the child explores new foods his friends introduce and may reject some of his old favorites that his playmates do not accept. Fortunately the schoolchild has a strong incentive to "grow big and strong" like his parents, older siblings, or favorite sports star.

Schedule meals around school hours. Occasionally, working mothers may serve hasty, skimpy breakfasts or no breakfast at all, which not only sends children off to school without proper energy and vitality for the day, but also paves the way for them to become adults who "just aren't hungry for breakfast." Avoid a very rushed schedule or undue excitement as much as possible, because disturbances dull a child's appetite.

124

Schoolrooms are great breeding grounds for communicable diseases. These illnesses usually decrease the appetite while increasing the child's nutritional needs to compensate for fever and infection. Hence, mother's ingenuity plays a decisive role as she turns an everyday salad into a clown's face, or a plain custard into a pleasant surprise by adding bits of bright-colored fruit. Necessary fruit juices go down much better with a flexible drinking straw.

The school-age child can eat almost anything an adult eats. Allow him a certain freedom of choice, however. Since every child arrives home from school "starved," mother should plan in advance a nourishing snack such as orange slices and oatmeal cookies rather than let the youngster raid the refrigerator.

Weight problems, either overweight or underweight, may predominate in the school-age child. The inactive child who nibbles all day long often grows overweight. Unfortunately the obese child tends to become the adult who battles the weight problem all his life. On the other hand, the nervous child may lose interest in food and subsequently lose weight. He then has no padding for his falls and more readily succumbs to illness.

Both problems need the cooperation of the parents. Encourage the nibbling child to limit his munching to regularly scheduled snacks of low-calorie vegetables, and his meals to the basic foods with fewer desserts. Encourage him to participate in outdoor activities and make the television set less prominent in family life. The underweight child may need supplemental feedings of milk drinks and other high-calorie foods to help him gain weight. Overemphasis on table manners may adversely affect the child's appetite.

**Teens**

One day, after parents have just stored away the high chairs and training bikes, they suddenly come face-to-face with a bewildering creation—a teen-ager. The teen-ager of thirteen is mostly child, and then, with varying stages of changes through the next few years, at nineteen he is mostly adult.

Teen years bring the second rapid growth spurt, which girls usually reach at ages twelve to fourteen and boys at ages fourteen to sixteen. Mothers who once begged and bribed a small boy to eat, now stand aghast as that same boy, now in his teens, eats three peanut butter and jam sandwiches, two apples, four cookies, a quart of milk, and then asks, "What's for dinner?" Not only do their bodies grow at an alarming rate, but they also undergo the stress and nervous strain of developing their personalities. They strive for independence. This accumulation of growth presents a nutritional challenge to meet the expanding needs of the young adult. While caloric needs soar along with the need for vitamins and minerals, and protein and fat, the untrained teen-age appetite, unfortunately, does not always crave nutritionally adequate food.

Alice Garrett Marsh describes this period in *Everyday Nutrition:* "Practically all teen-agers tend to have a few food service peculiarities to which they have a right. . . . They do not care too much for mixtures and casserole dishes. For the most part they like their foods separate. . . . A teen likes to have some informal meals to which he can come and go—especially when he has his mind on some special project. He likes food and eating with a minimum of fanfare."—P. 91.

Teen years give the young person a last chance for excellent body building. Boys, interested in muscles and body building, consciously consider the rewards of balanced meals. However, their appetites know no bounds, and they will eat almost anything and everything they can get their hands on, including "empty calories," such as candy bars, cake, soft drinks, shakes, etc. Wise mothers provide generous servings from the Four Food Groups to satisfy hunger and provide strong, vibrant bodies for their teen boys.

Teen-age girls are the most poorly fed of all age groups. Their greatest deficiencies are calcium and iron, since they most often exclude from their diet milk, eggs, vegetables, potatoes, and bread. The young lady, extremely weight and figure conscious, experiments with any fad diet, diet pill, and noncaloric food or beverage. Her eating habits fluctuate—one day indulging in French pastries and chocolate creams, and the next day eating only grapefruit and hard-boiled eggs so that she can squeeze into a new dress one and a half sizes too small. Her drive toward independence and her need to break away from family food patterns exceed her teen-age brother's. Her mind whirls with thoughts of dating, fashionable clothes, and popularity, rather than the beautiful woman nature intended her to be, capable of bearing healthy, vigorous babies at some future time.

Skin problems may erupt during the teen years. A well-balanced diet emphasizing fruits, vegetables (especially green and yellow), whole grains, milk, and sufficient water to help remove wastes, is the best dietary defense. Some foods, such as rich desserts, fats, chocolate, and nuts, seem to trigger acne. Low-fat milk helps control persistent acne.

Overweight may become a problem for young adults who limit their exercise to lying before the television or talking on the telephone for hours. Instead of carefully planning their caloric intake to match their growth and activity, the teen-ager's concept of weight control often consists of skipping meals (especially breakfast), omitting bread, milk, potatoes, and vegetables because they are "too fattening," then, ironically, snacking all day on soft drinks, candy, chips, and sweets. The breakfast skipper usually encounters a midmorning slump, thus reducing activity and inducing a sweet snack which dulls the appetite for lunch but wears off just in time to necessitate after-school munching. A large, late dinner tops off the day, and several bedtime snacks follow. Consequently, the overweight teen feels he gains weight even though he "hardly eats anything."

Quoting Mrs. Marsh again: "A food is a poor choice unless it satisfies some needs other than hunger. Does it furnish some protein for building? Does it supply some minerals, some vitamins? If it is soda pop, candy, or syrupy things, it does not. If it is rich desserts, the calories will be supplied in abundance and the other nutrients, though present, will be very low in amount. The wise teen will choose from real fruit or vegetable juice, milk drinks that are not overrich, crispy raw vegetables, and sandwiches of good-quality bread and nourishing fillings. Such foods build bodies, which cannot be said for sweet rolls or doughnuts and pop."—P. 91.

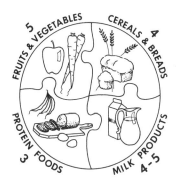

The Four Food Groups furnish the best eating pattern for teens. The servings of food recommended each day for teenagers are as follows:

Fruit and Vegetable Group _____ 5 servings
    2 servings which supply vitamin C
        (Citrus, tomatoes, cabbage, strawberries, etc.)
    1 serving of which supplies vitamin A
        (A very dark green or yellow vegetable)
Cereal and Bread Group _____ 4 servings
Protein Group _____ 3 servings
Milk Group _____ 4-5 servings
    (Weight watchers can use low-fat milk.)

"Parents have a special part in teen-age nutrition. In spite of the size of shoes, the sophistication of the clothes, the adult richness of the son's voice, the grown-up beauty of a daughter, the ability of both to do things, it is the parents' work to:
"Supply the food;
"Prepare the food;
"Serve the food in a good home climate.
"It does not mean that teens do not take on responsibilities of

many sorts. They can earn money, take on increasing amounts of home responsibilities, cook, clean, garden, farm, build, care for younger children. However, if the teen takes the responsibility of getting a good profession or trade, he or she must do so during the teen and young adult years.

"The responsibility of food, three times a day and seven days a week, should rest on the parents. Good nutritional advantages of the home and a creative home atmosphere are mainly the parents' work. Teens are not ready for such total responsibility. They are ready to become 'officers of the day,' first assistants and strong support to parents, but not to take parents' responsibilities.

"With parents fully responsible and definitely on the job in the fuller sense of homemaking, the teen-ager can be free to carry increasing responsibilities that prepare him for life. In the meantime, he can feel the support that he needs as he readies himself in education and daily experiences for a highly competitive world.

"Best of 'all, the young adult who has experienced good parental support during the teen years and into young adulthood has, in turn, a priceless preparation for his responsibility to his children. The children of today's successful family are tomorrow's parents with an 'inherited' blueprint for another successful home."—*Ibid.,* pp. 91, 92.

Chapter 11
## GOLDEN TOMORROWS


Modern medical advances have lengthened the life-span. The many discoveries relating to the cause of disease, the development of vaccines to prevent spread of disease, the building of well-staffed, well-equipped hospitals to care for the sick and injured, have again brought man to the anticipated life-span of threescore years and ten. These advances, as well as sociological changes, have made prominent the study of aging and geriatrics in medical fields and the study of the aged in sociology.

Though dreaded by all, all need not experience senility and disability. They do not necessarily result from the natural wear and tear of the body, but instead come about by improper use and care of the body. The golden years can originate pleasant glimpses of intellectual stimulations finally realized, enriching hobbies pursued for the first time, a lifelong wealth of experiences shared with a youthful friend, bewitching grandchildren bringing enchantment without strain of responsibility, and increasing leisure hours filled with travel, recreation, rest, and social activities. Truly, for the individual who has carefully followed a few simple principles of moderation and positive health, life can "begin at forty."

Good nutrition begun at birth and maintained through advancing years provides wonderful life insurance for the mature years, whereas the effects of poor food selection eventually appear. All too often, individuals falsely assume that since they have reached full growth, have passed the childbearing years, and have reduced their activities, they need not carefully watch their eating habits. How erroneous! Continued health and well-being depend largely on continued observance of the Four Food Groups. Malnutrition prevails among senior citizens because this period of life accentuates many physiological, psychological, and sociological problems. Adult bones still need liberal supplies of calcium to prevent osteoporosis; adult muscles still need protein of high biological value for good muscle tone; adult eyes still need adequate carotene to prevent night blindness; etc. Senior citizens should consider the importance of each individual Four Food Groups puzzle piece, although this is a time to minimize three-dimensional stacking.

Certain physiological changes occurring with age affect nutritional patterns. Since body processes decrease, and strain, tension, and physical activities decrease, calorie needs likewise decrease. Adults at their ideal weight at age twenty-five should not gain additional weight. Adding even as little as one pound a year finally results in the addition of twenty-five or thirty extra pounds, placing one in the obese category.

Some problems of degeneration affect eating habits of the older person. Increasing years may decrease sense of taste and smell so that food loses its appeal and appetite dulls. When dentures replace permanent teeth, chewing becomes difficult or nearly impossible if dentures do not fit well or remain in a tumbler on the nightstand a majority of the time. Slower digestive processes may mean more problems of abdominal distension or distress. Constipation is common.

Dietary patterns formed while young usually persist throughout life. In reality, it is too late to effect a major change in a body that has suffered the consequences of a lifetime of poor eating habits. However, correct eating patterns begun even in later years can provide satisfying rewards. Income, of course, can greatly affect food selections. Retirement usually means a small, fixed income that must somehow stretch to meet expenses and the rising cost of living. Transportation problems may necessitate infrequent trips to small neighborhood groceries where prices are unduly high. Incentive is lacking to prepare tasty meals, full of variety and interest for one or two persons whose appetites are less than par. It becomes increasingly easier to buy soft, easy to chew, starchy, and sweet foods which require little or no preparation and cost relatively little. Herein lies the excuse to live on toast and tea. Older people, who unconsciously seek the Fountain of Youth, often fall prey to faddish food ideas claiming vigor and renewed youth. Usually such exotic preparations, unappetizing diets, or expensive drugs only rob them of money they could more profitably spend on nourishing food.

The elderly should recognize, then modify or eliminate, their individual nutritional problems. Those who find that advancing years bring increasing pounds should remember that reduced activity demands reduced calorie intake. Although calorie level should decrease, nutrient level must not go below the recommended allowance provided by the Four Food Groups. A regular program of daily, moderate exercise means that the older person can continue enjoying the foods he has been accustomed to eating, but perhaps in slightly smaller portions. In addition to stimulating circulation and increasing the caloric expenditure to a small degree, exercise also promotes intestinal motility and may help solve the problems of gastrointestinal distress.

When the appetite wanes, select a colorful variety of textures and tastes and serve them attractively with tangy seasonings or zestful garnishes. Cheery place mats, lacy napkins, a clever centerpiece, or dainty stemware can make mealtime more enticing. Consulting a competent dentist often eases mastication problems, or, for those who still have a chewing problem, foods can be ground, finely chopped, or creamed or pureed in a blender. Although pureed vegetables may not appear attractive, they make appealing cream soups or casseroles. Pureed fruit is a delightful addition to pudding and gelatin, or a topping for ice cream and cereal. If the budget allows, junior foods afford a wide variety of delicious ready-to-eat chopped and pureed foods; serve them plain or add them to soup, puddings, sandwich spreads, and sauces.

For the increasingly slowing digestive process, eat at regular intervals small amounts of plain food without excess fat or seasonings. Those prone to intestinal distress should not eat rich sauces, heavy desserts, and fried or greasy foods. Strong-flavored vegetables such as onions, cauliflower, and legumes can produce abdominal distension if one limits exercise. Mild constipation in the elderly often results from inadequate fluid intake, lack of exercise, or a diet high in starch and low in fruit and vegetables. Stewed fruit, fruit juice (especially prune and fig juice), green vegetables, adequate fluids, along with regular exercise may alleviate this condition.

The effort to prepare two or three hot foods, a casserole of several ingredients, or baked products may seem wasted when a person lives alone. But where can one more wisely spend his time than in preserving his health? One can economize on cooking procedures with planning. A freezer or large freezing unit in a refrigerator especially helps a single person or a couple living alone, since multiple portions of a food can be prepared at one time and frozen in meal-size portions for a later date. For example, cook sufficient rice for (1) chop suey, (2) rice pudding, (3) rice and milk with brown sugar, (4) Spanish rice—all of which will appear on the menu during the next few weeks. If you do not own a freezer, you can successfully store some foods in the refrigerator for a few days after cooking, such as macaroni, part of which you could use in a casserole today and part in tomorrow's salad. The chapter "Artist at Work" offers many other helpful suggestions for meal planning.

A valuable appliance for the person preparing meals for one or two is the toaster oven. It heats rapidly and bakes small casseroles of two or four portions with less expense than would a regular-size oven. It can also double as a toaster and a broiler. An electric teflon frypan also heats rapidly to specified temperatures and allows one to prepare fried foods with a minimum of fat. It requires a small amount of space, sits on the table or counter for easy accessibility, and holds food at the table at a desired temperature for indefinite periods.

The mature person who has a wealth of experience to share

with his young friends may discover mealtime to be an ideal hour for socializing. Inviting friends, neighbors, or guests at church to share a simple meal adds incentive to again prepare tantalizing dishes. This is a time when favorite recipes can reappear, frequently to the surprise and delight of younger diners. However simple the meal, sharing it heightens the enjoyment.

With modern medical knowledge and positive health habits which include proper eating patterns, adults may look forward to advancing age as "Golden Tomorrows" full of vigor and productivity.

Chapter 12
## ENGINEERED CURVES

The overweight person encounters a variety of complex problems. He has a much greater chance of chronic illness, such as high blood pressure, heart disease, arthritis, diabetes, and liver and gallbladder disturbances. He may forfeit certain positions of employment because of his appearance and limited activity.

Why is nearly 30 percent of America's population overweight? Social activities encourage the eating of high-calorie desserts and snacks. After twenty-five years of age, body processes tend to slow down. Similarly, physical activity often diminishes as the person purchases more laborsaving devices for the home, advances in his job from manual and active labor to a more sedentary phase, and finds a car waiting in the driveway to take him on errands. Many people try to compensate for emotional problems by compulsive eating. Obesity itself is not inherited, but a parent can pass to his child poor eating habits.

The person who stops smoking notices a particular problem in gaining weight. Smoking dulls the senses of taste and smell, and the ex-smoker suddenly discovers the delicious flavors of food he has not really tasted since he began to smoke. In addition, he has the almost uncontrollable physical habit of reaching for something to put in his mouth.

The first step in reducing body weight is a visit to the doctor. He alone can determine the cause of weight gain and any physical problem or complication involved, and prescribe an acceptable reducing regimen of diet and coordinated exercise. The philosophy of weight reduction is to correct faulty eating patterns. Therefore, crash or fad diets may reduce weight temporarily, but at the same time they upset nutritional well-being. Since it is neither practical nor advisable to remain on such a regimen very long, the dieter quickly regains lost pounds when he resumes his normal eating habits.

Before successfully mastering overweight, a person needs to understand the cause of his weight problem. Realizing why a person craves rich desserts, why he has a compulsion to nibble, and what emotional need triggers overindulgence greatly simplifies reduction. Perhaps he must recognize his inactivity. Next, the individual should determine the desirable weight for his age, sex, height, and activity, and then keep an accurate record of his weight by weighing once a week on the same scales, at the same time of day, and wearing the same amount of clothes. Body weight normally fluctuates a little from day to day because of fluid retention or loss. Even those who do not need to lose weight should consult the scales regularly to watch for sudden, unaccountable weight loss, which may be the first indication of illness, or to guard against gaining more than five pounds above desirable weight.

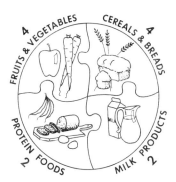

A wise reducing diet maintains the nutrition of the individual while reducing his weight. It consists of a reasonable variety of palatable, low-calorie everyday foods that give the feeling of well-being and yet cost little. It can be extremely simple. Almost any choice of the recommended adult servings from the Four Food Groups adds up to only 1,000 to 1,200 calories with needed nutrients in good supply. Most moderately active adults can lose weight on 1,200 calories a day.

Breakfast, an important meal for the weight watcher, should contain a good source of protein such as milk, eggs, vegetable protein foods, or peanut butter; this gives a feeling of satiety and decreases the midmorning slump, and consequently decreases the desire for a midmorning snack. People who say, "I am just not a breakfast eater," usually mean they have permitted themselves to acquire a bad habit. Perhaps they overeat in the evening and go to bed with a full stomach, thus dulling morning appetite. After an extra ten minutes in bed they must rush, and have no time to eat. The many quick breakfast possibilities make this a flimsy excuse since a nourishing breakfast is much more rewarding healthwise than ten more minutes of sleep.

Slow eating and thorough chewing may aid in losing weight. However, lingering at the table after finishing the meal can encourage second, third, or even fourth servings of tempting foods. A wide variety of food at a meal may invite the eater to have at least one serving of everything and consequently eat too much. Tension at mealtime may encourage rapid eating and second helpings to compensate for the uneasy feeling.

Sometimes the importance of coordinated exercise is neglected in a reducing program. Though calorie expenditure by specific exercise may not seem striking, regular moderate exercise benefits all age groups, and regular, appropriate exercise especially benefits the middle-aged or older individual. Such a program usually allows a person to eat a variety of food, including an occasional dessert. If you sensibly apply regular exercise, it will not harm you. Exercise improves muscle tone, stimulates circulation, gives a sense of well-being, and provides a release for emotional tensions that might otherwise lead to further indulgence in food. Walking, though a lost art, is one of the best exercises, since it involves many muscles and leaves the body in better muscle tone even hours later.

The overweight person may not overeat at meals, but may consume hundreds of calories in between meals. Nibbling plagues those who have stopped smoking, and the American way of life encourages snacking—the popularity of coffee breaks, the multitude of tantalizing snack foods which advertisers constantly keep in view, the drive-in restaurants on every corner, the vending machines in operation twenty-four hours a day, and the fact that everyone does it! Most adults would enjoy optimum health on two or three balanced meals a day and very few, if any, snacks. If you eat snacks, schedule them regularly and plan them in advance as a part of the allowed diet. Even though one realizes raw vegetables are a wise snack-food choice, potato chips, popcorn, candy, and such are much more accessible. So the determined dieter makes readily available a variety of freshly washed and pared vegetables such as carrots, celery, cucumbers, and tomatoes. Fresh fruit, used moderately, tomato juice and vegetable juice, dill pickles, and low-fat milk also provide good between-meal snack possibilities for overeaters.

Those wishing to reduce can usually eat regular food at home or in restaurants, keeping a few important facts in mind. Avoid large portions and second servings. You can eliminate without great nutritional loss such high-calorie foods as salad dressing, sauce, gravy, jam, jelly, preserves, fried or greasy foods, candy and sweets, soft drinks, rich desserts, and pastries. Foods you need not completely eliminate but should consume in very limited amounts are sugar, honey, molasses, butter, margarine, oil, shortening, and cream. Eat vegetables without additional amounts of butter or margarine; do not sweeten cereal; replace whole milk with low-fat or buttermilk; eat fruit either fresh or canned with little sugar or honey.

Motivation forms an essential part of successful weight reducing. Some people find striving for a reasonable goal in a specified space of time spurs them on to success. Group encouragement stimulates some, and weight charts help others. Placing a red check on the calendar each day the dieter holds to his resolutions may add incentive. Employ whatever motivates you to lose weight sensibly. Remind yourself with the words, "I choose to eat less."

The underweight individual may battle just as hard to attain desirable weight as does the overweight person. For him, also, correction of body weight depends on motivation and knowledge of food values.

Do not envy "skinny" people. The underweight have less resistance to infection and experience more fatigue. Underweight during pregnancy increases the likelihood of encountering complications. Adipose tissue is desirable in the right amounts for padding, for keeping the body warm, and for supplying energy stores in time of stress. Poor nutrition and underweight are often closely related.

The physician should determine the cause of underweight. It occurs most frequently and is most serious in youth, when the young body needs ample supplies of energy, protein, vitamins, and minerals. The underweight person is often tense and nervous, due in part to poor nutrition. Often he eats irregularly, selects poor foods, and has either a spasmodic or indifferent appetite. He may not receive adequate rest, which makes him more tense and nervous.

Since the diet of the underweight person often lacks essential nutrients, he should first of all change his eating patterns to conform to the recommended servings of the Four Food Groups. It is necessary to place special emphasis on the Protein Group, since body protein must be replaced as well as body fat. The underweight person may select freely from the "additions" mentioned on page 26. The increase in amount of food eaten should begin gradually, because a sudden overload of food may result in loss of appetite. Rapid weight gains usually increase adipose tissue only instead of coordinated gains of muscle, body protein, and body fat. A weight gain of two pounds per week is a reasonable goal. To facilitate this gain, add 400 to 800 calories a day above the amount needed to maintain body weight.

Determine desirable weight for the underweight person by means of charts stating correct weight for height, age, and sex. Regular weighing, once a week on the same scales, at the same time of day, wearing the same amount of clothing, is recommended as for the overweight person. Keeping an accurate weekly record of weight not only adds incentive but also aids in adjusting the diet to meet energy requirements.

Diet principles for the underweight oppose the diet principles for the overweight. Do not take low-calorie soups such as broth and bouillon, vegetable salads, vegetable juice cocktail, and beverages at the beginning of the meal as appetizers, since these fill the stomach without adding appreciable amounts of calories. Although foods from the Four Food Groups should constitute the main portion of the diet, additions of salad dressing, cream sauce, gravy, jams, some extra fat, whole milk or cream, cream soup, and reasonable amounts of desserts may facilitate weight gain. Reduce bulk in the diet in favor of foods high in caloric and nutritional value. Sometimes the following replacements can be made: tossed salad by marshmallow fruit salad with sour-cream dressing, asparagus spears by lima beans in cheese sauce, an egg omelet by cashew nut loaf with brown gravy, or a fresh fruit dessert by a fruit cobbler with whipped cream.

Regularly scheduled meals and snacks prepared attractively and appealingly, eaten in an unhurried, pleasant atmosphere, stimulate lagging appetites. Diet, often inadequate alone, coupled with regular exercise stimulates circulation, builds muscle tone, and often alleviates the underweight problem. Adequate rest lends a calm to the spirit and decreases the calories expended.

Maintaining desirable weight, being neither overweight nor underweight, is good life insurance. Correct improper weight by adjusting eating patterns to either decrease or increase calories while still maintaining high levels of necessary nutrients. Ideally, such a program of positive health begins during childhood with well-balanced meals, regular exercise, and adequate rest and recreation. The wise family schedules activities around such essentials. By weighing regularly, you can discover weight discrepancies early and alter them immediately while the problem is relatively simple and more easily corrected.

Chapter 13

# TEETH THAT LAST

An individual does not have pearly white teeth, even and free of fillings, as a matter of chance. They directly result from heredity, good nutrition, and daily care. Teeth break food into small particles that digestive juices and enzymes can act upon. Unless solid foods are masticated, the body cannot properly digest them or utilize the nutrients. The digestion of starches begins in the mouth when saliva mixes with food during the chewing process.

Because the foundation or basic structure of the tooth to a great extent determines its wearability, properly formed teeth with adequate nutrients resist decay. Tooth and bone structures begin growing about the seventh week of intrauterine life and necessitate generous supplies of protein, calcium, phosphorus, and vitamins A and D for pregnant women. Nutritional conditions prevailing during tooth formation, both before and after birth, affect tooth structure most. The infant at birth, although seemingly toothless, has nearly all of his deciduous teeth and several of his permanent teeth partly developed and, therefore, requires continued supplies of protein, calcium, and phosphorus found in milk. By the third month, fortify baby's milk diet with vitamins A and D to ensure healthy gums and teeth. According to the discretion of the physician, accomplish these additions by food additions or supplements.

Calcium and phosphorus are the chief mineral components of the tooth, and vitamins A, C, and D regulate the building process of these particular tissues. Even after the tooth forms, adequate supplies of calcium and phosphorus help prevent dental caries. During enamel formation and calcification, the daily ingestion of minute quantities of fluoride, taken either in fluoridated water or in supplemental drops or pills, makes the enamel decay resistant throughout life. The result of fluoride treatment is most effective when begun before the tooth buds erupt.

The inclusion of certain foods in the daily menu assures adequate amounts of the essential building materials. Milk supplies three of the nutrients needed for lasting teeth—protein, calcium, and phosphorus. Fortified milk furnishes vitamin D. Some vitamin-C-rich foods are citrus fruits, strawberries, and raw cabbage. Since not all people have the benefit of fluoridated water, fluorine may be prescribed in pill or liquid form. With the exception of fluorine, the simple Four Food Groups provide all nutrients necessary to ensure decay-resistant teeth.

Preserving teeth requires not only eating the right nutrients, but also including the right food textures in the diet. If you expect your teeth to last, put them to good use. Even during infancy the sucking action aids jaw development. Later, chewing develops and maintains strong teeth, jaws, and healthy gums. The average diet consists of two types of food textures: *detergent foods,* which sweep over, around, and between teeth and soft tissues; and *impacting foods,* which are soft and sticky, require little chewing, and adhere to the teeth. Apples, raw carrots, whole-wheat bread, and hard crusts are detergent foods, whereas mashed potatoes, white bread, jam, stewed prunes, and ice cream exemplify impacting foods. The average diet today contains too many soft foods to maintain healthy gums and teeth. Why not end each meal with a detergent food, then brush the teeth thoroughly? If you cannot brush after every meal, swish water between your teeth to remove much of the food and bacteria that otherwise adhere.

Dental caries are infections caused by cariogenic streptococci acting upon specific carbohydrates. Sucrose—table sugar—is the most highly cariogenic carbohydrate. Among the low cariogenic sugars are lactose (milk sugar), fructose, glucose, and sorbitols.

Especially in children's mouths, this cariogenic streptococcus grows easily and rapidly. Therefore, it is of prime importance to a child's dental health to limit the sucrose-containing foods in the diet, sticky sweets between meals, in particular. Dental caries are related more closely to the frequency with which carbohydrates, particularly sucrose, enter the mouth rather than to the total amount of carbohydrate consumed. Allowing the child to snack on sucrose-containing foods many times during the day greatly increases the risk of his developing dental caries. Snacks should not consist of empty calories—food high in sugar without protein, minerals, and vitamins. If snacks form part of the diet, choose them from the glorious array of fresh fruits and vegetables.

Teeth that last must be built in prenatal life. Good structures require good foundations built solidly from the ample storehouses of protein, vitamins, and minerals. Positive nutrition for a lifetime, daily hygiene with proper brushing, and professional dental supervision are required for teeth to last.

Chapter 14
## EMERGENCY STOPS


The main theme of ABOUT NUTRITION is preventive medicine and positive health through proper diet. It does not attempt
to prescribe diet therapy. However, we shall devote some space to
a brief discussion of heart disease—America's No. 1 health problem—and the relationship of diet to heart disease. Diet is only
one of several "risk factors" noted by the American Heart Association as contributing to the incidence of heart disease.

Followers of the Seventh-day Adventist health program have
considerably less *heart disease* than does the average American
person. One study suggests that Adventist men have 40 percent
less coronary artery disease than typical age-matched American
men, and Adventist women have 15 percent less coronary artery
disease than typical age-matched American women. Adult serum
cholesterol level of Adventists was found significantly lower
than that of an age-matched control group. The probable reasons for these finds are because in the typical lacto-ovo-vegetarian
diet, fat provides only 30 percent of the calories, and one third of
these are from polyunsaturates; and because of the avoidance of
caffeinated beverages, alcohol, and tobacco.

Lowering the total fat intake and the percentage of saturated
fat reduces the risk of heart attack. For a technical explanation
of saturated and unsaturated fat, see pages 35-46. Foods high in
saturated fats are meat and meat fats, butter, cream, whole milk,
whole-milk products, egg yolks, hydrogenated vegetable fat, and
coconut oil. Liquid vegetable-seed oils and margarines whose first
or second stated ingredient is liquid vegetable-seed oil are high in
polyunsaturates.

The American Heart Association recommends a fat intake of not more than 25 to 30 percent of total calories. This means, a 2,500-calorie diet should contain not more than 84.4 grams of fat daily. The average American diet includes a fat intake of 40 to 45 percent of total calories, and in most cases, Mr. Middle-class Businessman consumes 50 to 60 percent of his calories in fat.

In a practical vein, a typical 2,500-calorie diet might include these fat-containing foods:

| Food | Grams of fat |
|------|:---:|
| 2 cups whole milk | 18 |
| 3 ounces steak, beef | 24 |
| 2 ounces luncheon meat, ham | 10 |
| 3 teaspoons margarine | 18 |
| 3 tablespoons coffee cream | 9 |
| 1 tablespoon mayonnaise | 12 |
| 1 piece apple pie | 15 |
| | 106 |

106 grams fat x 9 calories per gram = 954 calories from fat (954 is 38.16 percent of 2,500).

With this list as the *only* source of fat for the day, this 2,500-calorie diet contains 38.16 percent of total calories derived from fat—dangerously above the recommended level.

The lacto-ovo-vegetarian who eats 2,500 calories a day could substitute gluten for the steak and spun soy protein for the luncheon meats and come within safe limits. Using the same fat-containing foods with these substitutions, the list appears like this:

| Food | Grams of fat |
|------|:---:|
| 2 cups whole milk | 18.0 |
| 3 ounces Choplet | .05 |
| 2 ounces Wham | 5.8 |
| 3 teaspoons margarine | 18.0 |
| 3 tablespoons coffee cream | 9.0 |

| 1 tablespoon mayonnaise | 12.0 |
| 1 piece apple pie | 15.0 |
| | 77.85 |

77.9 grams fat x 9 calories per gram = 701 calories from fat (701 is 28 percent of 2,500.)

With this list as the *only* source of fat for the day, this 2,500-calorie diet contains 28 percent of total calories derived from fat —within the recommended level.

After lowering total fat intake, next lower the percentage of saturated fat by substituting liquid vegetable-oil products for meat and dairy fat whenever possible. The lacto-ovo-vegetarian diet eliminates meat fats, so we shall consider only dairy fats.

| *Common sources of saturated fat* | *Possible replacements* |
|---|---|
| 1. Whole milk | 1. Low-fat milk |
| 2. Butter and margarine | 2. Margarine whose first or second ingredient is liquid vegetable oil |
| 3. Vegetable shortening | 3. The above margarine or liquid vegetable oil |
| 4. Cream and nondairy creamers* | 4. Powdered skim milk or low-fat milk |
| 5. Cottage cheese, cream cheese, yellow cheese | 5. Dry cottage cheese, skim-milk cream cheese and cottage cheese, Farmers' cheese, Hoop cheese |
| 6. Chocolate | 6. Cocoa |
| 7. Ice cream and milk sherbet | 7. Ice milk, fruit ice |
| 8. Butter cake and cookies | 8. Oil cake and cookies, angel cake, sponge cake |

Along with these replacements, limit certain foods such as doughnuts, chips and snack crackers, egg yolks, salad dressings,

---

*So-called nondairy creamers, although lacking in cream, are made with coconut oil, which is as saturated as dairy cream.

most commercially made cake, chocolate and cream candies, cookies, and pastries. This does not mean that the average person should never eat foods containing saturated fat, but these foods must not appear often on his menu or in more than small amounts.

The lacto-ovo-vegetarian diet also reduces cholesterol intake, which now appears less important than saturated fat and total fat intakes. Cholesterol is found only in animal fats—meat fats, dairy fats, and egg yolks. Eliminating meat fats and using limited amounts of dairy fats and egg yolk place the cholesterol intake within the recommended level.

Daily use of caffeine has come to the attention of doctors and nutritionists as another possible factor in raising the risk of coronary disorder. Caffeine affects the nervous system in a way resembling physical or emotional stress. It stimulates the adrenal gland to produce extra epinephrine, which, in turn, causes the heart to beat faster and speeds up many other body processes. For a short time this gives a person a feeling of more energy. It lifts only temporarily, however, and more coffee must be taken to continue the effect.

"Is this stimulation harmful in any way?" People react in very different ways to caffeine. Those accustomed to drinking large amounts of coffee often notice fewer effects from it than do those who do not use it regularly. Research seems to indicate that, in any case, this repeated stimulation and stress do burden the heart and eventually lower its resistance to heart attacks and other types of damage.

In many cases, the use of coffee closely accompanies an increase in the lipid fat levels of the blood similar to the increase noted in association with emotional stress or a diet high in sugar and saturated fat.

It is easy to see that the continual stress caused by routine coffee use might work together with increased blood lipid levels to account for the observation that the coffee drinker more readily succumbs to heart disease than the person who uses little or no coffee.

These are but a few of the factors involved in reducing the risk of heart attack. Obesity, lack of exercise, smoking, heredity, high sucrose intake, excess sodium intake—all seem to take their toll. Because heredity is a fixed risk factor, it is of vital importance that the individual control those "risk factors" that he can control by an overall good and sensible diet. Dietary control that puts the *amount* and *type* of fat in its right perspective should begin early in life. It is an overall control that demands care in food purchasing, food preparation, and eating habits, and that joins with other controls of appropriate exercise and elimination of habits that destroy good health.

Even the most hearty who practice excellent nutritional habits occasionally succumb to the ever-present multitude of viruses and germs. Right habits of eating before, during, and after illness strengthen the body, facilitate recovery, and help protect it from future diseases. Dietary suggestions follow for the person suffering from minor short-term illnesses. For chronic or more serious illnesses, consult a physician promptly, and carefully follow any special diet recommended by a physician.

*Colds* are a common malady, and as yet no real remedy has been found for a cold except to rest, to drink large quantities of fluids, and to treat the symptoms. Often, the counsel to "drink plenty of fluids" or to "force fluids" may not be easy to follow. How much is plenty? Six to eight cups of fluid daily are desirable under normal conditions, so an increased fluid intake may mean two and a half quarts and more daily.

This fluid intake may consist of a variety of things besides water, such as soups, broth, fruit juice, vegetable juice, fruit ices, gelatin, milk and milk drinks, herb tea, and cereal beverages. Mothers who must "force fluid" for toddlers may find the use of gaily-colored straws, individual-sized fruit-juice cans, popsicles, and multicolored gelatin cubes in tall parfait glasses helpful. Allowing a "small fry" to pour his own juice from a small, unbreakable pitcher or freeze his own colored ice cubes can make mother's job less difficult.

*Fever*—an elevation of temperature above normal—warns that

148

something is amiss in the body. Report high or continued fevers to a physician for treatment. During fever important changes affecting nutrition are a sharp elevation in metabolic rate, increased protein metabolism, and accelerated loss of body water and certain minerals through increased urinary output and perspiration. Therefore, increase caloric intake to compensate for the increased metabolic rate, supply liberal amounts of high biological protein, and increase fluid intake. The old adage "feed a fever" has merit.

Foods that will supply calories, fluids, and some proteins to the fever patient are fruit juices with gelatin, milk shakes, custards, milk puddings, cocoa beverages, ice cream, cereal with cream and sugar, and cream soups.

*Vomiting* may accompany many minor illnesses. Repeated vomiting can quickly dehydrate a child or an individual who has taken very little fluid in the past few hours. Sometimes vomiting can be stopped by taking teaspoonfuls of hot tea for its astringent effect. Do not withhold fluid so that the "stomach may rest," but administer it in sips in the form of ice chips, ginger ale, water, teas, and diluted fruit juice. Always report severe or continued vomiting to a physician.

*Constipation,* the difficult passage of feces, is not uncommon, as is evidenced by the high expenditures for laxatives each year and the multiplicity of such products available. Normal evacuation varies with the individual. The most important factor for good health is to maintain elimination at intervals suitable for comfort whether it be twice a day, every day, or every third day. Lack of sufficient fluids, lack of exercise, nervous strain, or a diet low in fiber and high in refined foods may precipitate temporary constipation. Overuse or long-continued use of laxatives and enemas, poor personal hygiene, resisting the urge to defecate, or failing to take time for regular evacuation may cause more serious constipation.

To correct temporary constipation, allow regular time for elimination, eat regular meals, receive adequate rest, exercise to stimulate motility, take at least eight to ten cups of fluid a day, and include bulk in the diet such as whole grains in bread and cereal, raw fruit, stewed fruit with skins, and raw vegetables such as celery sticks, tossed salad, carrots, and cabbage. Spastic constipation does not respond to this treatment and requires specific medical treatment for each case.

*Diarrhea*—frequent, fluid stools—often occurs with a minor illness. In severe or prolonged diarrhea consult a physician, since dehydration or electrolyte imbalance may suddenly occur. Mild diarrhea may diminish with the use of a liquid diet plus smooth cereals. Encourage liquids to compensate for the excessive fluid loss. Bananas, boiled skim milk, and apple pectin found in apple juice and fresh apples (scraped) may aid in eliminating the symptoms.

Illnesses signal prompt attention. Consult professional medical aid if symptoms do not respond quickly to rational home treatment. The ill individual may or may not desire to eat. In most minor disorders, to miss a meal or two, or even a whole day of meals, is not traumatic. It is very necessary, however, to take fluids regularly each day, especially when fever, vomiting, and diarrhea occur. Good nutrition should be continuous as far as possible, and must not be interrupted for long periods in the very young and in the elderly.

## SECTION IV

# On Your Guard

Chapter 15

# POISON IN THE POT

Some attractively prepared and served foods may be unsafe to eat. Invisible toxic agents that give no warning of their presence by flavor, odor, or appearance cause food poisoning. Hours, or even days, after eating a toxic food, sickness or death may strike. Food poisoning occurs one of three ways: (1) from toxic substances occurring naturally in food, (2) from bacteria in food, or (3) from toxins produced by bacteria living in food.

## Food Toxins

The toxic substances occurring naturally in plants and animals receive comparatively little attention today. In past ages, man discovered by trial and error which "foods" caused sickness and death. Such items cannot be purchased in grocery stores. Owing to constant surveillance by the Food and Drug Administration, this country's food supply is wholesome and reliable. Foods that do not meet government standards are quickly removed from the market. The *FDA Papers* publish monthly the reports of such recalled items and of the Food and Drug Administration's continuing search for safer and improved foods.

Although the foods purchased are reliable, some toxic plants grow in every area of the country and may be obtained through channels other than the grocery store. Anyone involved with food preparation needs to know naturally occurring toxins.

Many varieties of mushrooms are poisonous—some so deadly that merely handling one, then touching the fingers to the mouth, can transfer a fatal amount of toxin. Since several of the edible mushrooms have poisonous "look-alikes," no one but an expert with adequate experience should decide which are edible. Consumers not qualified to select wild mushrooms should use only those grown commercially. Several types of mold and fungus related to mushrooms may grow on otherwise edible foods and cause poisoning. Never eat dry grains, nuts, corn, legumes, or any food that shows evidence of mold.

Certain raw foods contain toxic substances which heating inactivates. Common examples are soybeans and lima beans. These legumes are entirely safe after cooking. The fava bean, whether cooked or raw, has frequently been reported to cause poisoning in individuals sensitized to it.

Solanine is a toxic agent in immature or sprouting potatoes. Cut away green areas on potatoes, for they contain solanine. Rhubarb leaves can cause illness because of a concentration of oxalic acid, whereas the young stems can be eaten without harm.

Some persons fear "can poisoning" from commercially canned foods refrigerated in their opened cans. The can will not cause poisoning; however, it may impart a metallic flavor to the food after opening, caused by the reaction of food acids and air on the metal can. Tomatoes and tomato juice commonly develop a metallic flavor from opened cans, which, although not poisonous, certainly does not add to palatability.

Occasionally, foods are poisoned by substances that get into them by mistake. Store separately and clearly label all cleaning supplies, insecticides, or any nonfood items kept in the kitchen. Always store such nonfoods out of the reach of youngsters.

Somewhat obliquely related to food poisoning is the question occasionally raised concerning the radioactive contamination of food. With increased use of radioactive materials, the government agencies who protect food supplies continually monitor the level of radioactive materials in food. Milk is frequently used as an index, for the cow forages over large areas and could ingest quantities of radioactive compounds. The fact that milk is used as a reference food, and is occasionally associated with radioactivity in reports, does not make it any less safe than other foods subject to radioactive contamination.

## Bacterial Food Toxins

The more common form of food poisoning results from bacterial contamination of food. Bacteria, like man, require various nutrients for their growth; thus the more nutritious combinations provide excellent media for bacterial growth. The living bacteria themselves, or the toxins produced by bacteria, may cause food poisoning.

Various bacteria of the genera Salmonella and Streptococcus cause poisoning by infecting the host. Staphylococcus organisms produce toxins which cause poisoning. Within two to forty-eight hours after ingestion of these bacteria or their toxins the symptoms of poisoning may occur: nausea, vomiting, abdominal cramps, and diarrhea. Death from such poisoning is rare; complete recovery usually takes one to three days. Severe cases may require hospitalization, where fluids and electrolytes (mineral salts) lost by vomiting and diarrhea are replaced intravenously to prevent dehydration and mineral imbalance.

For poisoning by these bacteria to occur, four conditions must exist:

1. Food providing an excellent nutrient media for rapid bacterial growth.

Foods upon which these bacteria vegetate are those rich in protein and carbohydrates, often in combinations such as cold meat salad, potato salad, cream puddings and pies, custards, stuffed eggs, and cream puffs. Since acid ingredients slow bacterial growth, add lemon juice to potato salad, egg salad, and protein sandwich fillings.

2. Inoculation of the bacteria into the food.

This occurs easily in many ways. The food handler may contaminate the food by unwashed hands that have touched pimples or come in contact with intestinal excreta, or hands that have even a small infection on them; by droplets from talking or coughing over food when the handler has an infected throat; or by tasting from a stirring spoon or licking the fingers. (Poisoning by Staphylococcus organisms is most commonly introduced

155

in these ways.) Never use hands for mixing foods, especially those foods that you do not heat before serving. It is also the food handler who likely contaminates foods with Salmonella. Only rarely and under "dirty" conditions does the disease originate from rodent, fly, or cockroach contact with the food, or from a diseased animal providing the food. If a cow or hen is infected by Salmonella, pasteurization of the milk and at least soft boiling of the egg destroy all Salmonella organisms.

3. Room temperature.

With nutrient material available, bacteria multiply very rapidly at room temperature. Refrigeration temperatures delay their growth, but only after the entire mass of food has cooled. For prompt cooling, thinly spread foods that readily support bacterial growth. Freezing stops bacterial multiplication but does not kill the organisms. When frozen foods thaw, the bacteria again become active, and precautions must be taken to prevent their growth.

4. Sufficient time for bacterial growth.

Under the proper conditions, bacteria can multiply sufficiently within two to three hours to cause poisoning. Every food handler should assume foods like those mentioned in item No. 1 have been inoculated, and either serve them immediately before bacteria can multiply, or refrigerate or freeze the food to prevent multiplication. Never allow these foods to remain at room temperature.

Botulism is another type of food poisoning caused by toxins produced by living bacteria. This poisoning is dealt with individually because it is unique in several ways.

*Clostridium botulinum* spores are common and not harmful. Only when they remain alive in airtight containers and are not destroyed by heat do they produce a deadly toxin. One taste from a jar infected with growing botulism organisms could supply a fatal dose of the toxin, which attacks the nervous system rather than the gastrointestinal tract. Fatigue, visual disturbances, and muscular paralysis lead to death from respiratory muscle failure. Whereas the other types of bacterial food poisoning rarely kill, botulism poisoning kills approximately 65 percent of those infected.

Toxins of C. *botulinum* are not formed in a distinctly acid media, which includes most fruits. The most common source of this poisoning is home-canned vegetables (green beans, corn, beets, spinach, asparagus) and home-canned meats or sea foods. C. *botulinum* spores are present in the soil in many areas, and thus may remain on subacid foods when canned. The spores withstand boiling temperatures, then begin to grow inside the sealed jar. When the jar is later opened, no physical change in the food appears, yet one taste of the food may result in death.

To make home-canned foods safe follow these precautions:

1. Pressure-can subacid foods (vegetables, meats, and meat analogues) according to pressure and timetables published by reliable sources. (Ball Brothers Company, Incorporated, Muncie, Indiana. Kerr Field Service Department, Sand Springs, Oklahoma. United States Department of Agriculture, Home and Garden Bulletins.) Only pressure-canning heats the food sufficiently above boiling temperatures to kill the spores which could later produce the toxin.

2. Boil home-canned, subacid vegetables for ten minutes before tasting or serving. Sufficient boiling renders foods safe if poisoned with the toxin. Even so, nonpressure-canning of subacid foods is not recommended. One thoughtless taste could kill.

3. Freezing or commercial canning renders subacid foods safe.

It is imperative for safety that all food handlers are educated to the existence of the unseen microorganism world. A classic example to the contrary is the uninformed housewife who, in the days before really cold refrigeration, placed yesterday's potato salad on the table while telling her friend of vague digestive tract upsets and sickness that had troubled her family frequently that summer. The friend, eyeing the potato salad, suggested maybe their trouble was food poisoning. The housewife replied in a huff, "I don't put poison in my food!"

To be sure prepared foods are safe, remember the following points: Promptly serve or quickly refrigerate all high-nutrient foods that are handled or are in close contact with people and remain uncooked. In refrigerating such food, spread it three inches or less in depth and leave uncovered until thoroughly chilled. "High risk" foods such as potato salad, egg salad, and meat sandwiches should not be served at picnics or in lunches unless the people furnishing these foods understand how to handle them. Thoroughly chill such foods immediately after preparation, and then hold them not more than two hours out of refrigeration. Never bring unused foods conducive to the growth of bacteria home from picnics. Pressure-can all subacid foods, then, when opened, boil thoroughly before tasting.

Individuals involved in food handling must know that what they prepare is completely safe. If there is the slightest question as to the safety of a food, adopt the motto, "When in doubt, throw it out!"

Chapter 16
## CURRENT QUACKERY

Today's sophisticated consumer smiles when he reads accounts of uninformed old-timers who fell prey to the nutritional quackery vendors of the "good ole days." Mystical snake oils, wolf milk, or cure-all tonics sold under the flicker of torches and to the beat of drums, promising relief of ills and revitalization of life, were purchased. After finishing the entertaining article, this same intelligent American will likely include costly vitamin pills or food supplements with his dinner. This educated individual is convinced that supplements or specially grown foods prevent subclinical deficiencies which he feels sure will result from eating inadequate foods grown on depleted soil, and which processing further devitalizes.

This sophisticated, intelligent consumer is only today's version of yesterday's snake-oil buyer, now fallen prey to a laboratory-coated charlatan who dispenses the same quack diets and fake supplements that promise a shortcut to health. By a clever blending of science with superstition and a smattering of pseudoscientific terms, the propagandist can easily persuade and present apparently plausible theories which promise much.

The individual likely to fall into faddism can usually be classed in one of four categories: (1) those who adopt new ideas and diet systems from fashion rather than concerning themselves with the facts behind the ideas, (2) those who worry about their state of health and feel there must be some way to make their current good health better, (3) those with real illnesses who find it easier to believe bizarre claims of a quack than ethical medical advice, (4) neurotic individuals who derive psychological reas-

159

surance from following an unusual diet plan. Eating uncommon or even disliked foods comforts these individuals.

The food faddism racket costs ten million Americans $500 million a year. Every report indicates food quackery is continuing to rise despite the efforts of regulatory agencies and educational programs. Many faddish notions are relatively harmless health-wise. They merely relieve one of his money and are ridiculous when viewed through the scientific eye. But when promoters claim cures for diseases or symptoms not caused by a dietary deficiency at all, or when one follows the fad cure instead of getting proper medical attention, tragic results can follow.

Many fad diets restrict their followers to a few rather unusual or exotic foods. The human body needs a variety of nutrients which a variety of common foods best supplies. Often the faddist keeps in relatively good health by "fad-hopping." Fad diets can grow very monotonous, which luckily drives the faddist to try new systems. A grapefruit diet one week, yogurt and molasses the next, followed by a raw carrot and hard-boiled egg jag may ultimately furnish the needed nutrients to prevent nutritional deficiencies, although it is far from an ideal dietary pattern.

Due to mass communication devices and educational accomplishments, the American consumer is very health conscious. Low-calorie foods, polyunsaturated fats, trace minerals, minimum daily requirements—all are terms used in everyday conversation. The consumer is constantly made aware of important nutritional advancements, but he rarely has the specialized knowledge necessary to distinguish between nutritional sense and nonsense.

The advice of self-styled nutritionists, over-zealous salesmen, best-selling so-called nutrition books, or the more subtle advertising gimmicks need not bewilder. To put himself in control, the consumer needs to become an informed skeptic—informed on factual guidelines, and skeptical of any person or product that does not measure up to ethical standards.

**Evaluating the Source**

*Believe* it if the information came from:

The American Dietetic Association.

The American Institute of Nutrition.

The American Society for Clinical Nutrition.

U.S. Department of Agriculture and The Food and Drug Administration.

State Departments of Health.

University Nutrition Departments.

Nutrition sections of the following scientific groups:

The American Medical Association.

The American Public Health Association.

The American Home Economics Association.

Individuals who have an academically recognized degree in nutrition or dietetics, such as the Registered Dietitian.

*Beware* if the advice is from:

Someone with something to sell.

That a large portion of the American public will accept doorbell "doctors" or mailed circulars as the last word on nutrition is amazing. Question the authority of anyone with a product to sell. (Do not confuse this point with fully qualified persons employed by an ethical food or equipment company, who give correct information about nutrition or the product's use.

One posing under authoritative titles (doctor, professor, nutritionist, biochemist) but who lacks credentials necessary to support such a title.

Quickly discredit the "Authority" if he claims accepted scientific organizations persecute him. No amount of piety can replace true competence. The intelligent individual must watch out for quotations from reputable nutrition authorities which someone takes out of context or warps to suit his own ends.

161

A person who is a professional in another field, but not in nutrition.

> Educated individuals may be authorities in their area, but possessing an advanced degree in another area does not make one a nutrition authority.

A well-meaning but uninformed friend.

> Personal testimonies are a most believable promotional gimmick. They may cleverly sell a product, or your friend may *sincerely* believe what he says. The fact remains that all the sincerity in the world does not make a false idea true.

Popular books on nutrition.

> Many of them contain some good information mixed with misinformation. Frequently they contain medically and nutritionally unsound advice. Such books are dangerous and unsuitable for reference.

### Evaluating the Information

*Do not believe* it if:

It guarantees exuberant health or everlasting youth.

It blames all ill health entirely on poor nutrition.

It says foods lack nutrients because of depleted soil or overprocessing.

It recommends any one "miracle food" or "loaded" formula.

A reducing program allows you to eat anything you desire.

It offers a cure for a condition that ethical medical science thus far has been unable to remedy.

It is straight misinformation, such as:

> "Grape juice constitutes a good source of vitamin $B_{12}$."
> "The composition of avocado and milk is similar. Use avocado in the place of milk."
> "Honey is a food; refined sugar is a poison."
> "Arrowroot flour has a high calcium content."

162

Outright false statements are frequently the most difficult to recognize unless the doubter is trained in nutrition or has a reliable source of information. False statements are commonly made in regard to the composition of foods. Every interested individual should have a reliable food composition booklet. Then when a self-styled nutritionist appears, or a new cookbook says honey is a good source of minerals, or almonds can be made into a milk substitute, the composition reference will show these claims are completely erroneous. Two excellent sources for reliable compositions of foods are the Home and Garden Bulletin, No. 72, with foods listed in common serving portions, or the U.S. *Department of Agriculture Handbook, No. 8*, which lists foods in 100-gram and one-pound portions.

When evaluating diet systems for reducing, gaining, or a myriad of other reasons, the most reliable guide is: Do they measure up to the Four Food Groups without warping the picture? Overemphasis or exclusion of any one group signals a nutritional imbalance. A nonfortified beverage made from soybeans belonging to the protein group cannot replace foods in the milk group. You cannot ignore the cereal group just because you wish to eat only an abundance of fruit. All foods have been assigned their position in one of the Four Food Groups according to their nutrient content. Wishing a food into another group will not change its nutritive contribution to the diet.

The most reliable guide to remember when confronted with a "miraculous" potion is: No one food or supplement is the key to good health. The human body needs the correct balance of nutrients, and common foods best furnish these. The swindler may claim that any number of vague aches and pains, fatigue or nervousness, are due to something lacking in the diet which his special dietary food or capsule will absolutely cure. "True, $22.99 a month, but when the family's *health* is at stake, money should be of no concern," he cajoles. By gulping loaded pills and potions without a physician's direction, the gullible are likely to incur imbalances which could never occur if they ate common foods as outlined by the Four Food Groups. For instance, a continuous overdose of vitamin A or D can lead to hypervitaminosis—a serious toxic condition, especially if children or expectant mothers are the victims.

The following chapter lists some of the more commonly believed fallacies along with explanations of the nutritional facts.

Chapter 17
# FOOD FADS AND FACTS

Many faddish ideas spring from nutritional facts warped to suit someone's personal motives. Just the right amount of truth blended with the erroneous, along with a slight play on the emotions, and the charlatan has built a very convincing story and probably a lucrative business. The following are examples of commonly encountered fallacies with explanations of the facts.

✔American soil is so impoverished that our foods lack nutrients.

Neither poor soil nor rich soil affects the composition of plants and their seeds or fruits. The quality of the soil definitely affects the crop yield, but not its nutritional quality. Plants need certain elements for growth and reproduction and simply will not grow if the required elements are not available. Different strains of the same food plant may vary somewhat in nutrient content due to genetic variations. For example, different varieties of oranges develop slightly different amounts of vitamin C. Because of this fact, food composition listings from different sources will show some variations. New strains of food plants are constantly developed, such as corn higher in lysine and tomatoes with more vitamin C. The genetic code, not soil fertility, determines the composition of a plant.

Iodine deficiency is the only condition that may result from exclusively eating foods grown where the soil lacks iodine. Such areas in the United States are the Great Lakes states and Northwestern states. Sufficient iodine is easily obtained in deficient areas by using iodized salt.

✔Mono- and diglycerides come from animal sources and can be added to fats labeled as "pure vegetable."

Mono- and diglycerides may be derived from either animal or vegetable sources. Chemically speaking, they are related to fats and may be considered partially digested fats. Enzymes in the intestinal tract break each fat molecule (Figure 1, below) by a stepwise process, first into a diglyceride (Figure 2) and one fatty acid, then into a monoglyceride (Figure 3) and two fatty acids, and finally into an alcohol (glycerol) and three fatty acids (Figure 4), which the body absorbs.

The chemist can "digest" animal or vegetable fats in the laboratory to produce mono- and diglycerides. The source of these pure chemical entities need not be stated according to law. They are added in extremely small amounts (usually around one tenth

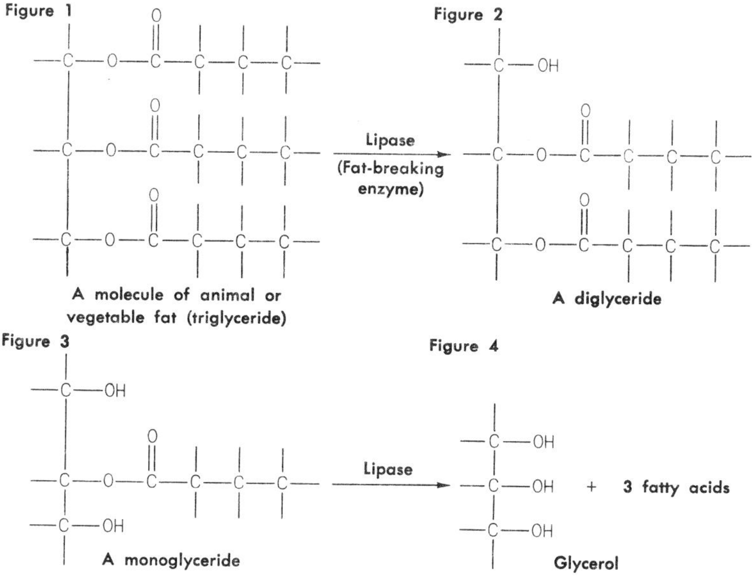

Figure 1

A molecule of animal or vegetable fat (triglyceride)

Lipase (Fat-breaking enzyme)

Figure 2

A diglyceride

Figure 3

A monoglyceride

Lipase

Figure 4

Glycerol

+ 3 fatty acids

of 1 percent) to margarine and butter to make the product more spreadable.

✔Pesticides poison our foods. Chemical food additives are dangerous.

When foods are grown without protection, healthy bugs and a decreased crop result. Without some means of control, food-crop pests would cause incalculable damage every year, resulting in a scarcity of food and increased costs. When pesticides and other chemical preparations are properly applied and the harvest is carefully washed before eating, man derives no harmful effect. The federal government has set tolerance limits which they carefully check. If pesticide residues in foods exceed these limits, the foods cannot be sold.

Food additives have received a great deal of attention from food manufacturers and consumers. Those who have no knowledge of chemistry tend to become emotional at the thought of chemicals in their food. Yet every item in our world is a chemical or a mixture of chemicals: flowers, the Mackinac Bridge, food, and cells in the human body.

Certain additives benefit, such as vitamins and minerals added in carefully regulated amounts. Additives such as emulsifiers and stabilizers may not benefit the consumer but facilitate processing. Spoilage retardants increase keeping ability and provide food the consumer expects at prices he can afford. In many ways food additives are responsible for the superior selection and quality of the foods we enjoy. Without them it would be impossible to feed the mass American population.

Before a food processor receives permission to use an additive, it must be proved safe by biological testing. Food additives are under constant study by the federal government, private agencies, and educational centers, and after passing government standards for safety, study on the additives' long-term effects continues. If such research shows extended use or cumulative amounts to be harmful, the additive is removed from the approved list.

Dr. Harvey W. Wiley, a founder of the present Food and Drug Administration that is directly responsible for consumer protection, made a guiding statement in 1867 that seems to stand as the FDA's motto and is quoted in each issue of the *FDA Papers*: "We are carefully to preserve that life which the Author of nature has given us, for it was no idle gift."

✔Organically grown foods are superior to chemically fertilized foods.

Food crops need certain nutrients for growth just as do human beings. The plant cares not whether the elements it draws from the soil came from decomposing organic matter or from a sack of "chemical" fertilizer. All nutrients are chemical compounds. Nitrogen is nitrogen, iron is iron, sodium is sodium—its source does not matter, only whether it is present or lacking in the soil. If certain nutrients are scarce, the crop yield will be small but nutritionally equal to lush crops grown in rich soil. Large-scale crop-nutrient needs can best be met by commercially prepared fertilizers. Without current-day knowledge of soils and the use of all types of fertilizers, this nation's food-crop yield would greatly diminish and food prices would skyrocket.

✔Cooking or commercial processing destroys the nutritive value of foods.

Many a food cultist promotes a diet totally composed of foods in their natural state. Although some raw fruits and vegetables are desirable, the human digestive system is not constructed to handle great quantities of raw materials as the grazing animal's digestive system can. The body more easily and completely digests properly cooked foods; thus we derive greater nutritive value from them. Modern food-processing methods quick-freeze or can fruits and vegetables at their peak nutritional value.

Some consider white flour, refined cereals, or any number of other processed foods devoid of nutritional value. However, enrichment can nutritionally improve foods that lost nutrients through extensive processing. Enriched cereal products have had thiamine, riboflavin, niacin, and iron replaced to correspond with the food's original nutritional level.

🖙One must eat raw foods, nuts, or sprouts for their enzymes.

Cooking temperatures inactivate enzymes—complex specks of nonliving proteinous matter. Plants and animals produce hundreds of different enzymes for their very specialized needs. Plant enzymes help bring about maturity and ripening. The enzymes essential to human life function in digestion, absorption, metabolism of foods, and building and repair of cells. Living cells excrete each enzyme to perform its very specific function. Enzymes produced within our own bodies cannot be interchanged. Digestive enzymes secreted into the digestive tract could never replace the enzymes needed to handle foodstuff once it is in the bloodstream. Our bodies cannot adopt the enzymes in raw plant foods. The best to be said of plant enzymes is that they are harmless. The body digests the eaten enzymes and may utilize the microscopic bit of protein. Every living organism makes all its own enzymes to fit all its own needs.

🖙Natural vitamins are better than synthetic vitamins. Everyone should take vitamins.

A vitamin is a chemical compound with a specific structure. Hand an analytical biochemist a laboratory-produced "synthetic" vitamin sample and an extracted "natural" vitamin sample, and he would not find any difference between the two. Structure and function identify a vitamin; its origin makes no difference.

Not everyone should take vitamins. Concentrated vitamin preparations should be considered medicine and taken only under a physician's direction. Self-medication may be only a costly waste or may lead to serious toxic conditions. The body cannot store water-soluble vitamins (vitamin C and most of the B vitamins) for the simple reason that they dissolve in water, and excesses are excreted. Taking an overabundance of these vitamins wastes money. However, the body stores the fat-soluble vitamins (especially vitamins A and D), which may lead to the toxic condition of hypervitaminosis. Hypervitaminosis is frequently a conundrum. Symptoms of the condition may resemble the deficiency symptoms of the vitamin involved. Both too little and too much vitamin A or D may result in poor growth, nausea, diarrhea, itching skin, or headache. If you follow the Four Food Groups, you will never get in toxic amounts the vitamins and minerals naturally present in foods.

➤ Eating hard fats will raise the cholesterol level, and this may cause heart attacks.

Consumption of hard animal fats or hard (hydrogenated, saturated) vegetable fats does tend to increase the blood cholesterol level. An elevated blood cholesterol level may be one factor leading to coronary heart disease, and moderate changes in food selection can reduce the amount of cholesterol in the bloodstream. First, the average American should cut down on fat intake, then replace hard fats with small amounts of seed oils or products made from these nonhydrogenated oils (high in polyunsaturates).

Cholesterol is a normal, useful body constituent originating from synthesis within the body and from foods. Conforming to a very strict "cholesterol-free" diet may cause considerable inconvenience to the individual besides those near and dear, and may result in little or no change in blood cholesterol levels, because of the body's ability to make cholesterol.

An elevated cholesterol level is not the only cause of heart attack. High blood pressure, overweight, too little physical activity, cigarette smoking, tensions and stresses, eating largely of simple carbohydrates (all sugars and honey), diabetes, and heredity are all risk factors. An individual can reduce or eliminate these risk factors, with the exception of heredity, if he so chooses.

➤ Honey is high in minerals and will not cause tooth decay. Refined sugar is a poison; raw sugar is a food.

A brief table clearly compares the various forms of sugar:

| | | Calories | Calcium mg. | Iron mg. |
|---|---|---|---|---|
| White sugar | 1 tablespoon | 45 | 0 | tr. |
| Honey | 1 tablespoon | 65 | 1 | 0.1 |
| Corn syrup | 1 tablespoon | 60 | 9 | 0.8 |
| Brown sugar | 1 tablespoon | 50 | 12 | 0.5 |
| Molasses, light | 1 tablespoon | 50 | 33 | 0.9 |
| Molasses, blackstrap | 1 tablespoon | 45 | 137 | 3.2 |

Honey poorly supplies minerals, especially when one considers the number of calories it contains. As for not causing tooth decay, honey's mixture of sucrose, fructose, and glucose does not differ from any other sugar in that respect. Any sugar in the mouth encourages bacterial growth, which in turn produces decay-causing substances.

White sugar (sucrose) is refined from cane and beets by man. Honey is also a refined product. The bee drinks nectar, concentrating and changing it from its original form before placing it in the comb. The only real choices between these two forms of sugar are (1) whether the individual prefers either man or bees to have concentrated this high-calorie food, and (2) the taste difference. One advantage of honey might be its greater flavor and sweetness, thus tiring the taste buds more quickly than would white sugar, and one might eat less.

Refined sugar is raw sugar with the molasses removed, brown sugar is refined sugar with a controlled amount of the molasses returned to the sugar. Whether the sweetness comes in granular or syrupy form, or in dark or light color, it is still sugar—a simple carbohydrate and a concentrated calorie source one should limit in the diet. Although blackstrap molasses does contain considerable amounts of minerals, it cannot be considered a common mineral source. The average individual consumes very little blackstrap molasses in a year's time, and appreciable amounts irritate the gastrointestinal tract.

171

🖊Avocado "milk" furnishes the same nutrients as cow's milk and can be used in its place. Almond "milk" can be made for children.

The only substance legally termed "milk" is the secretion of the mammary gland. Milk is a superb blend of nutrients manufactured to meet the very exacting needs of the growing mammal. Avocado or almonds or any other fruit or nut made into "milk" can never exactly replace milk. In terms of protein alone, no single plant protein is completely balanced in the essential amino acids necessary for growth. A correct mixture of different vegetable proteins can furnish all the essential amino acids, but when nuts, seeds, or avocado make up the majority of the mixture, the fat (and calorie) content becomes prohibitive. Milk makes an especially important contribution to the body's calcium and phosphorus needs. The body best absorbs and utilizes these two minerals when eaten in approximately a one-to-one ratio, which milk closely provides. Milk is definitely superior to fruit or nut preparations during the months of life when growth and development largely depend upon a formula food.

|  | Cal. | Pro. gm. | Fat gm. | Ca. mg. | Phos. mg. | $B_1$ mg. | $B_2$ mg. | Niacin mg. |
|---|---|---|---|---|---|---|---|---|
| Whole milk, 1 cup | 160 | 9 | 9 | 288 | 227 | .08 | .42 | 0.1 |
| Avocado (½), 123 grams | 160 | 2 | 14 | 12 | 52 | .13 | .24 | 2.0 |
| Almonds, ¼ cup | 212 | 6 | 19 | 83 | 46 | .08 | .33 | 1.2 |

🖊Homemade or "health" baking powders are better than commercial preparations. Alum and lime are harmful substances sometimes included in commercial baking powder.

A baking powder combines an edible acid and alkali with

a drying ingredient which helps prevent moisture from accumulating, thus causing the two to react and loose carbon dioxide prematurely. The acid and alkali portions must be very precisely weighed and combined so that each reacts totally with the other (stoichiometrically balanced) leaving no alkaline or acid residue. Commercial baking powders can be more carefully produced with precision equipment so that they are stoichiometrically balanced and leave only a neutral residue. Home measuring of baking powder components lacks precision and leaves true balancing of ingredients to chance. An excess of alkali (soda) leaves an alkaline residue which destroys B vitamins and irritates the digestive tract.

The so-called "health" baking powder, available under several common brand names, is a calcium phosphate product. The body can use the neutral calcium phosphate salt left in the food after baking.

Alum is not harmful. Many of our foods contain aluminum salts. The idea that aluminum injures began somewhere in the dusty past during trade wars between competitive baking powder companies and competitive cooking utensil companies. The fact that this idea is totally unfounded has not dulled its popularity over the years. Lime is another name for calcium oxalate—calcium is essential to life.

✔Milk and sugar ferment in the stomach to produce alcohol.

If milk and sugar produced alcohol in the stomach, few would patronize the beer and wine industries. Any individual wishing to go on an alcoholic binge could do so just by eating these very available and inexpensive foods. Likewise, anyone not wanting to wash his problems away in alcohol would become drunk from merely eating food. A few extremely rare individuals have hosted abnormal gastrointestinal bacteria which could produce alcohol from food, and they remained in a drunken stupor most of the time until medical science could eradicate the unusual microorganisms.

Sugar is classed chemically as an alcohol, as are many of

173

our foodstuffs. These food alcohols and alcohols resulting from normal digestion do not cause inebriation.

Fermentation means the decomposition of a substance into simpler substances. Sugar does "ferment" during the normal process of digestion, for it is broken down into simpler sugars. Fermentation could also be an acidic fermentation, which, in this case, does not result in the formation of alcohol.

Possibly the fact that sugar is classed as an alcohol, or a misconception of the word *fermentation*, has led to the erroneous idea that sugar ferments in the stomach to produce inebriating alcohol.

🖊Alcohol is formed as yeast dough rises.

True. Fallacy enters when persons become concerned that some lingers when the bread is eaten.

For optimum growth yeast requires sugar, moisture, and a warm temperature. The tiny yeast plants utilize sugar if it is present in the dough, or they can produce an enzyme capable of converting some of the starch of flour into sugar. As the yeast multiplies, it produces carbon dioxide gas, causing the dough to rise. Some ethyl alcohol also results. This alcohol is very volatile, and the heat of the oven rapidly drives it off. No alcohol remains in baked bread.

Scientific advancements in crop propagation, storage, and transportation have blessed our country with a great variety of nutritious foods. The individual can meet his nutritive needs by eating readily available, inexpensive foods. If a person happens to like the flavor of yogurt, wheat germ, carrot juice, or sprouted alfalfa and has the extra time and money to supply himself with these less-common foods, he should be allowed to eat them in moderation without being classed as a faddist. But when an individual eats these rather unusual foods to the exclusion of more common ones, or when he thinks the unusual foods nutritionally superior, he has become a faddist. Faddish beliefs are especially hurtful when they lead one to buy costly specialty foods or home-size processing equipment out of a limited budget and in place of good food. Common foods abundantly furnish all the nutrients needed. The reward for eating these common foods according to the Four Food Groups puzzle is excellent nutritional health. Correct nutrition provides the best insurance in all stages of life.

Chapter 18
# IN REVIEW

This book presents a way of life that includes the use of all good food. Normal nutrition ensues only when the food adequately supplies all nutrients. Good health follows good nutrition. Poor health inevitably results from poor nutrition.

Normally, undernutrition will not happen when one chooses his daily diet from ordinary foods according to the pattern of the Four Food Groups. Neither will overnutrition cause toxicity. The puzzle is easily put together. Each day as the homemaker or food service manager chooses from the four groups of food, she utilizes the metaphysics of the ages and the biochemistry of this century to feed each person. Each individual fed is most fortunate that he lives where food is available, when nutrition has become a well-understood science, and with someone who cares enough to provide food that nourishes the body for its best function and longest duration. He can with dexterity and confidence walk the tight rope of good nutrition—enough of all the good nutrients he needs, but not too much to unbalance the perfect metabolic processes of the human body.

The nutrients discussed throughout the book come from good, everyday food. Food comes from the field, garden, orchard, and dairy, or for most people from the various markets. Each person feeding himself or others should consider it a privilege to learn the principles of good food preparation in order to preserve nutrients, while he readies the food in the most acceptable form for life at its best.

With so many foods and varieties of foods from which to choose, everyone should become a scientist to the extent that he knows how to utilize the sciences vital to life. He should become an artist to the extent that the science of living is also an art. Then the science and art of eating should take only their rightful place as a part of life, supporting the spiritual and intellectual facets that involve life in its highest sense of values.

# Food and Nutrition Board, National Academy
## Recommended Daily Dietary
Designed for the maintenance of good nutrition

| | AGE [2] (years) From / Up to | WEIGHT (kg.) (lbs.) | HEIGHT (cm.) (in.) | kcal | PROTEIN (gm.) | FAT-SOLUBLE VITAMINS VITAMIN A ACTIVITY (IU) | VITAMIN D (IU) | VITAMIN C ACTIVITY (IU) |
|---|---|---|---|---|---|---|---|---|
| Infants | 0-1/6 | 4　9 | 55　22 | kg × 120 | kg × 2.2[5] | 1,500 | 400 | 5 |
| | 1/6-½ | 7　15 | 63　25 | kg × 110 | kg × 2.0[5] | 1,500 | 400 | 5 |
| | ½-1 | 9　20 | 72　28 | kg × 100 | kg × 1.8[5] | 1,500 | 400 | 5 |
| Children | 1-2 | 12　26 | 81　32 | 1,100 | 25 | 2,000 | 400 | 10 |
| | 2-3 | 14　31 | 91　36 | 1,250 | 25 | 2,000 | 400 | 10 |
| | 3-4 | 16　35 | 100　39 | 1,400 | 30 | 2,500 | 400 | 10 |
| | 4-6 | 19　42 | 110　43 | 1,600 | 30 | 2,500 | 400 | 10 |
| | 6-8 | 23　51 | 121　48 | 2,000 | 35 | 3,500 | 400 | 15 |
| | 8-10 | 28　62 | 131　52 | 2,200 | 40 | 3,500 | 400 | 15 |
| Males | 10-12 | 35　77 | 140　55 | 2,500 | 45 | 4,500 | 400 | 20 |
| | 12-14 | 43　95 | 151　59 | 2,700 | 50 | 5,000 | 400 | 20 |
| | 14-18 | 59　130 | 170　67 | 3,000 | 60 | 5,000 | 400 | 25 |
| | 18-22 | 67　147 | 175　69 | 2,800 | 60 | 5,000 | 400 | 30 |
| | 22-35 | 70　154 | 175　69 | 2,800 | 65 | 5,000 | - - | 30 |
| | 35-55 | 70　154 | 173　68 | 2,600 | 65 | 5,000 | - - | 30 |
| | 55-75+ | 70　154 | 171　67 | 2,400 | 65 | 5,000 | - - | 30 |
| Females | 10-12 | 35　77 | 142　56 | 2,250 | 50 | 4,500 | 400 | 20 |
| | 12-14 | 44　97 | 154　61 | 2,300 | 50 | 5,000 | 400 | 20 |
| | 14-16 | 52　114 | 157　62 | 2,400 | 55 | 5,000 | 400 | 25 |
| | 16-18 | 54　119 | 160　63 | 2,300 | 55 | 5,000 | 400 | 25 |
| | 18-22 | 58　128 | 163　64 | 2,000 | 55 | 5,000 | 400 | 25 |
| | 22-35 | 58　128 | 163　64 | 2,000 | 55 | 5,000 | - - | 25 |
| | 35-55 | 58　128 | 160　63 | 1,850 | 55 | 5,000 | - - | 25 |
| | 55-75+ | 58　128 | 157　62 | 1,700 | 55 | 5,000 | - - | 25 |
| Pregnancy | | | | +200 | 65 | 6,000 | 400 | 30 |
| Lactation | | | | +1,000 | 75 | 8,000 | 400 | 30 |

[1] The allowance levels are intended to cover individual variations among most normal persons as they live in the United States under usual environmental stresses. The recommended allowances can be attained with a variety of common foods, providing other nutrients for which human requirements have been less well defined. See text for more-detailed discussion of allowances and of nutrients not tabulated.

[2] Entries on lines for age range 22-35 years represent the reference man and woman at age 22. All other entries represent allowances for the midpoint of the specified age range.

| WATER-SOLUBLE VITAMINS | | | | | | | MINERALS | | | | |
|---|---|---|---|---|---|---|---|---|---|---|---|
| ASCOR-BIC ACID (mg.) | FOLA-CIN[3] (mg.) | NIA-CIN (mg.) equiv[4] | RIBO-FLAVIN (mg.) | THIA-MIN (mg.) | VITA-MIN $B_6$ (mg.) | VITA-MIN $B_{12}$ ($\mu$g.) | CAL-CIUM (g.) | PHOS-PHORUS (g.) | IODINE ($\mu$g.) | IRON (mg.) | MAG-NESIUM (mg.) |
| 35 | 0.05 | 5 | 0.4 | 0.2 | 0.2 | 1.0 | 0.4 | 0.2 | 25 | 6 | 40 |
| 35 | 0.05 | 7 | 0.5 | 0.4 | 0.3 | 1.5 | 0.5 | 0.4 | 40 | 10 | 60 |
| 35 | 0.1 | 8 | 0.6 | 0.5 | 0.4 | 2.0 | 0.6 | 0.5 | 45 | 15 | 70 |
| 40 | 0.1 | 8 | 0.6 | 0.6 | 0.5 | 2.0 | 0.7 | 0.7 | 55 | 15 | 100 |
| 40 | 0.2 | 8 | 0.7 | 0.6 | 0.6 | 2.5 | 0.8 | 0.8 | 60 | 15 | 150 |
| 40 | 0.2 | 9 | 0.8 | 0.7 | 0.7 | 3 | 0.8 | 0.8 | 70 | 10 | 200 |
| 40 | 0.2 | 11 | 0.9 | 0.8 | 0.9 | 4 | 0.8 | 0.8 | 80 | 10 | 200 |
| 40 | 0.2 | 13 | 1.1 | 1.0 | 1.0 | 4 | 0.9 | 0.9 | 100 | 10 | 250 |
| 40 | 0.3 | 15 | 1.2 | 1.1 | 1.2 | 5 | 1.0 | 1.0 | 110 | 10 | 250 |
| 40 | 0.4 | 17 | 1.3 | 1.3 | 1.4 | 5 | 1.2 | 1.2 | 125 | 10 | 300 |
| 45 | 0.4 | 18 | 1.4 | 1.4 | 1.6 | 5 | 1.4 | 1.4 | 135 | 18 | 350 |
| 55 | 0.4 | 20 | 1.5 | 1.5 | 1.8 | 5 | 1.4 | 1.4 | 150 | 18 | 400 |
| 60 | 0.4 | 18 | 1.6 | 1.4 | 2.0 | 5 | 0.8 | 0.8 | 140 | 10 | 400 |
| 60 | 0.4 | 18 | 1.7 | 1.4 | 2.0 | 5 | 0.8 | 0.8 | 140 | 10 | 350 |
| 60 | 0.4 | 17 | 1.7 | 1.3 | 2.0 | 5 | 0.8 | 0.8 | 125 | 10 | 350 |
| 60 | 0.4 | 14 | 1.7 | 1.2 | 2.0 | 6 | 0.8 | 0.8 | 110 | 10 | 350 |
| 40 | 0.4 | 15 | 1.3 | 1.1 | 1.4 | 5 | 1.2 | 1.2 | 110 | 18 | 300 |
| 45 | 0.4 | 15 | 1.4 | 1.2 | 1.6 | 5 | 1.3 | 1.3 | 115 | 18 | 350 |
| 50 | 0.4 | 16 | 1.4 | 1.2 | 1.8 | 5 | 1.3 | 1.3 | 120 | 18 | 350 |
| 50 | 0.4 | 15 | 1.5 | 1.2 | 2.0 | 5 | 1.3 | 1.3 | 115 | 18 | 350 |
| 55 | 0.4 | 13 | 1.5 | 1.0 | 2.0 | 5 | 0.8 | 0.8 | 100 | 18 | 350 |
| 55 | 0.4 | 13 | 1.5 | 1.0 | 2.0 | 5 | 0.8 | 0.8 | 100 | 18 | 300 |
| 55 | 0.4 | 13 | 1.5 | 1.0 | 2.0 | 5 | 0.8 | 0.8 | 90 | 18 | 300 |
| 55 | 0.4 | 13 | 1.5 | 1.0 | 2.0 | 6 | 0.8 | 0.8 | 80 | 10 | 300 |
| 60 | 0.8 | 15 | 1.8 | +0.1 | 2.5 | 8 | +0.4 | +0.4 | 125 | 18 | 450 |
| 60 | 0.5 | 20 | 2.0 | +0.5 | 2.5 | 6 | +0.5 | +0.5 | 150 | 18 | 450 |

[3] The folacin allowances refer to dietary sources as determined by *Lactobacillus casei* assay. Pure forms of folacin may be effective in doses less than one fourth of the RDA.
[4] Niacin equivalents include dietary sources of the vitamin itself plus 1 mg. equivalent for each 60 mg. of dietary tryptophan.
[5] Assumes protein equivalent to human milk. For proteins not 100 percent utilized factors should be increased proportionately.

# BIBLIOGRAPHY

**Books**

*New Cook Book.* Better Homes and Gardens. Des Moines, Iowa: Meredith Corporation, 1968.

BLAKESLEE, A., and STAMLER, J., *Your Heart Has Nine Lives.* Pocket Books. Englewood Cliffs, New Jersey: Prentice-Hall, Inc., 1963.

BOGERT, L. J., et al., *Nutrition and Physical Fitness.* 8th edition. Philadelphia: W. B. Saunders Company, 1966.

BURTON, B. T., *Heinz Handbook of Nutrition.* 2nd edition. New York: McGraw-Hill, Inc., 1965.

DIEHL, H. S., *Tobacco and Your Health: The Smoking Controversy.* New York: McGraw-Hill, Inc., 1969.

EASTMAN, N. J., *Expectant Motherhood.* 4th edition. Boston: Little, Brown, and Company, 1963.

*Family Cook Book.* Minneapolis, Minnesota: Pillsbury Publications, 1963.

*Handbook of Food Preparation.* Revised edition. American Home Economics Association, 1964.

KINDER, F., *Meal Management.* 3rd edition. New York: Macmillan and Co., Ltd., 1968.

KRAUSE, M. V., *Food, Nutrition and Diet Therapy.* 4th edition. Philadelphia: W. B. Saunders Company, 1966.

LEVERTON, R. M., *Food Becomes You.* 3rd edition. Ames, Iowa: Iowa State University Press, 1965.

LOWENBERG, M. E., et al., *Food and Man.* New York: John Wiley and Sons, Inc., 1968.

MAYER, J., *Overweight: Causes, Cost and Control.* Englewood Cliffs, New Jersey: Prentice-Hall, Inc., 1968.

MOWRY, L., *Basic Nutrition and Diet Therapy for Nurses.* 3rd edition. St. Louis, Missouri: C. V. Mosby Company, 1966.

MICKELSEN, O., *Nutrition, Science and You.* New York: Scholastic Book Services, Scholastic Magazine, 1964.

PROUDFIT, F. T., and ROBINSON, C. H., *Normal and Therapeutic Nutrition*. 13th edition. New York: Macmillan and Co., Ltd., 1967.

ROBINSON, C. H., *Basic Nutrition and Diet Therapy*. New York: Macmillan and Co., Ltd., 1965.

SONNENBERG, L., editor, *Everyday Nutrition for Your Family*. Los Angeles, California: Seventh-day Adventist Dietetic Association, 1960.

STARE, F. J., *Eating for Good Health*. Garden City, New York: Doubleday and Company, Ltd., 1964.

United States Department of Agriculture, *Composition of Foods*. Handbook No. 8. Washington, D.C.: U.S. Government Printing Office, 1963.

United States Department of Agriculture, *Food*. Yearbook of Agriculture. Washington, D.C.: U.S. Government Printing Office, 1959.

United States Department of Agriculture, *Food for Us All*. Yearbook of Agriculture. Washington, D.C.: U.S. Government Printing Office, 1969.

WHITE, E. G., *Counsels on Diet and Foods*. Washington, D.C.: Review and Herald Publishing Association, 1946.

WHITE, E. G., *The Ministry of Healing*. Mountain View, California: Pacific Press Publishing Association, 1942.

WILLIAMS, S. R., *Nutrition and Diet Therapy*. St. Louis, Missouri: C. V. Mosby Company, 1966.

WOHL, M. G., and GOODHART, R. S., *Modern Nutrition in Health and Disease*. 4th edition. Philadelphia, Pennsylvania: Lea and Febiger, 1968.

**Journals**

BELLET, S., et al., "Effect of Coffee Ingestion on Adrenocortical Secretion in Young Men and Dogs," in *Metabolism*, December, 1969, pp. 1007-1012.

BELLET, S., et al., "Effect of Coffee Ingestion on Catecholamine Release," in *Metabolism*, April, 1969, pp. 288-291.

BELLET, S., et al., "Response of Free Fatty Acids to Coffee and Caffeine," in *Metabolism*, August, 1968, pp. 702-707.

CHRISTAKIS, G., et al., "Effect of the Anti-Coronary Club Program on Coronary Heart Disease Risk-Factor Status," in *Journal of the American Medical Association*, November 7, 1966, pp. 597-604.

COONS, C. M., "Fatty Acids in Foods," in *Journal of the American Dietetic Association*, 1958, pp. 242-247.

HODGES, R. E., et al., "Dietary Carbohydrates and Low Cholesterol Diets: Effects on Serum Lipids of Man," in *American Journal of Clinical Nutrition*, February, 1967, pp. 198-208.

INGELFINGER, F. T., "For Want of an Enzyme," in *Nutrition Today*, September, 1968, pp. 2-10.

INGELFINGER, F. T., "Gastrointestinal Absorption," in *Nutrition Today*, March, 1967, pp. 2-10.

KERSHBAUM, A., "Tobacco Smoking and Atherosclerotic Vascular Disease," in *Malattie Cardiovascolari*, Vol. 8, No. 1, 1967, pp. 31-49.

KEYS, A., "Blood Lipids in Man—A Brief Review," in *Journal of the American Dietetic Association*, December, 1967, pp. 508-516.

PAUL, O., et al., "A Longitudinal Study of Coronary Heart Disease," in *Circulation*, July, 1963, pp. 20-31.

PAUL, O., "Stimulants and Coronaries," in *Postgraduate Medicine*, September, 1968, pp. 196-199.

RAAB, W., "The Nonvascular Metabolic Myocardial Vulnerability Factor in 'CHD,'" in *American Heart Journal*, November, 1963, pp. 685-706.

WALDEN, R. T., et al., "Effect of Environment on the Serum Cholesterol-Triglyceride Distribution Among Seventh-day Adventists," in *American Journal of Medicine*, Vol. 36, pp. 269-276.

WYNDER, E. L., et al., "Cancer and Coronary Artery Diseases Among Seventh-day Adventists," in *Cancer*, Vol. 12, 1959, pp. 1016-1028.

**Bulletins and Leaflets**

*FDA Papers,* Food and Drug Administration, Washington, D.C.

"Food for Fitness: A Daily Food Guide," United States Department of Agriculture, Agricultural Research Service.

Food and Nutrition Board: "Recommended Dietary Allowances," 7th revised edition. National Academy of Sciences, National Research Council Publication 1694, 1968.

Leaflets on Fat-Controlled Diets, American Heart Association, New York, New York.

"Nutrition, Diet and the Teeth," United Fresh Fruit and Vegetable Association, Washington, D.C. May, 1968.

"Nutrition in Old Age," United Fresh Fruit and Vegetable Association, Washington, D.C. October, November, and December, 1968.

"Nutritive Value of Foods," United States Department of Agriculture, Home and Garden Bulletin No. 72, 1970.

"Some Aspects of Food Preservation," Ball Brothers Company, Muncie, Indiana.

"Ten Short Lessons in Canning and Freezing," Kerr Field Services Department, Sand Springs, Oklahoma.

# SUGGESTED READING FOR SECTION I

*Basic Nutrition and Diet Therapy*, by Corrine H. Robinson.
*Eating for Good Health*, by Frederick J. Stare.
"Food," United States Department of Agriculture *Yearbook*, 1959.
*Food and Man*, by Miriam E. Lowenberg, E. Neige Todhunter, Eva D. Wilson, Moira C. Feeney, and Jane R. Savage.
*Food Becomes You* (3rd edition), by Ruth M. Leverton.
"Food for Us All," United States Department of Agriculture *Yearbook*, 1969.
*Meal Management* (3rd edition), by Faye Kinder.
*Nutrition and Diet Therapy*, by Sue R. Williams.
*Nutrition and Physical Fitness* (8th edition), by L. Jean Bogert, George M. Briggs, and Doris H. Calloway.
*Nutrition, Science and You*, by Olaf Mickelsen.
*Overweight: Causes, Cost and Control*, by Jean Mayer.
*Your Heart Has Nine Lives*, by Alton Blakeslee and Jeremiah Stamler.

(See Bibliography for publishers.)

## SELECTED READING REGARDING DIETARY FATS AND BLOOD LIPIDS

"Blood Lipids in Man—A Brief Review," by Ancel Keys, in *Journal of the American Dietetic Association,* December, 1967.

"Dietary Carbohydrates and Low Cholesterol Diets: Effects on Serum Lipids of Man," by R. E. Hodges, W. A. Krehl, D. B. Stone, and A. Lopez, in *The American Journal of Clinical Nutrition,* February, 1967.

"Effect of the Anti-Coronary Club Program on Coronary Heart Disease Risk-Factor Status," by George Christakis, in *Journal of the American Medical Association,* November 7, 1966.

Leaflets on Fat-Controlled Diets, The American Heart Association, New York, New York.

*Your Heart Has Nine Lives,* by Alton Blakeslee and Jeremiah Stamler.

(See Bibliography for publishers.)